Step by Step
Pediatric Echocardiography

Step by Step
Pediatric Echocardiography

Third Edition

Rani Gera

MBBS MD (Pediatrics)
Consultant
Safdarjung Hospital
Vardhman Mahavir Medical College
New Delhi, India

Foreword
HPS Sachdev

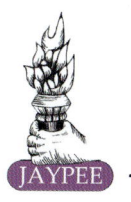

JAYPEE *The Health Sciences Publisher*

New Delhi | London | Philadelphia | Panama

Jaypee Brothers Medical Publishers (P) Ltd

Headquarters

Jaypee Brothers Medical Publishers (P) Ltd
4838/24, Ansari Road, Daryaganj
New Delhi 110 002, India
Phone: +91-11-43574357
Fax: +91-11-43574314
Email: jaypee@jaypeebrothers.com

Overseas Offices

J.P. Medical Ltd
83 Victoria Street, London
SW1H 0HW (UK)
Phone: +44-2031708910
Fax: +44 (0)20 3008 6180
Email: info@jpmedpub.com

Jaypee Medical Inc
The Bourse
111 South Independence Mall East
Suite 835, Philadelphia, PA 19106, USA
Phone: +1 267-519-9789
Email: jpmed.us@gmail.com

Jaypee Brothers Medical Publishers (P) Ltd
Bhotahity, Kathmandu, Nepal
Phone: +977-9741283608
Email: Kathmandu@jaypeebrothers.com

Jaypee-Highlights Medical Publishers Inc
City of Knowledge, Bld. 237, Clayton
Panama City, Panama
Phone: +1 507-301-0496
Fax: +1 507-301-0499
Email: cservice@jphmedical.com

Jaypee Brothers Medical Publishers (P) Ltd
17/1-B Babar Road, Block-B, Shaymali
Mohammadpur, Dhaka-1207
Bangladesh
Mobile: +08801912003485
Email: jaypeedhaka@gmail.com

Website: www.jaypeebrothers.com
Website: www.jaypeedigital.com

© 2015, Jaypee Brothers Medical Publishers

The views and opinions expressed in this book are solely those of the original contributor(s)/author(s) and do not necessarily represent those of editor(s) of the book.

All rights reserved. No part of this publication may be reproduced, stored or transmitted in any form or by any means, electronic, mechanical, photocopying, recording or otherwise, without the prior permission in writing of the publishers.

All brand names and product names used in this book are trade names, service marks, trademarks or registered trademarks of their respective owners. The publisher is not associated with any product or vendor mentioned in this book.

Medical knowledge and practice change constantly. This book is designed to provide accurate, authoritative information about the subject matter in question. However, readers are advised to check the most current information available on procedures included and check information from the manufacturer of each product to be administered, to verify the recommended dose, formula, method and duration of administration, adverse effects and contraindications. It is the responsibility of the practitioner to take all appropriate safety precautions. Neither the publisher nor the author(s)/editor(s) assume any liability for any injury and/or damage to persons or property arising from or related to use of material in this book.

This book is sold on the understanding that the publisher is not engaged in providing professional medical services. If such advice or services are required, the services of a competent medical professional should be sought.

Every effort has been made where necessary to contact holders of copyright to obtain permission to reproduce copyright material. If any have been inadvertently overlooked, the publisher will be pleased to make the necessary arrangements at the first opportunity.

Inquiries for bulk sales may be solicited at: jaypee@jaypeebrothers.com

Step by Step Pediatric Echocardiography

First Edition: **2004**

Second Edition: **2010**

Third Edition: **2015**

ISBN 978-93-5152-661-2

Printed at Replika Press Pvt. Ltd.

Dedicated to

*My daughters
Prerna and Akriti*

FOREWORD

Pediatric cardiology is generally viewed as a complex subject by practicing pediatricians. An important reason for this feeling is the fact that most of them have not been exposed to the intricacies of relevant technological advances in the field. Amongst various such techniques, echocardiography is used most frequently. This simple, noninvasive and inexpensive test has withstood the test of time and has proved invaluable for optimal patient management.

The first and second editions presented the essentials of the subject in a lucid and simplified manner. The simple step approach for performing echocardiography proved useful and was welcomed by the beginners. Of particular utility were the salient echocardiographic findings that were explained by illustrative sketches and highlighted text.

Following the success of the earlier edition, the author has labored exhaustively to bring out an enlarged and an updated third edition. Important additions include chapters on Fetal Echocardiography, Neonatal Echocardiography and Echocardiography in Intensive Care Unit. Apart from improved illustrations and production quality, another value addition is the inclusion of images encountered in the routine clinical practice.

HPS Sachdev
MD (Pediatrics) FIAP
Ex-President
Indian Academy of Pediatrics
Consultant
Sitaram Bhartia Institute of
Science and Research
New Delhi, India

PREFACE

Pediatric echocardiography is coming up in a major way, because of an increased awareness of early diagnosis and management of congenital heart diseases, especially the life-threatening ones. Pediatric echocardiography technique, though simple, requires a trained pediatric echocardiographer. It is an uncomplicated, noninvasive and low-cost technique providing a correct hemodynamic status of the heart, thus reducing the requirement of cardiac catheterization, which is invasive and expensive. With the advancement of technology, three-dimensional and four-dimensional echocardiography has been introduced. This has improved the technique to identify congenital or acquired heart disease, also having its functional implications. Hence, cardiac catheterization is used for the more complex cardiac conditions, and those requiring interventions and surgery. Also, with the introduction of functional echocardiography, the use of echo in intensive care units has increased, as its use in monitoring critically ill patients has proved beneficial. We acknowledge Dr Romit Saxena for his contributions to the chapter of Echocardiography in Intensive Care Unit.

Rani Gera

CONTENTS

Chapter 1. **Introduction** — 1

Chapter 2. **Position of the Patient and Transducer** — 11

Chapter 3. **M-Mode and Doppler Examination** — 24
M-mode 24
Doppler echocardiography 29

Chapter 4. **Echocardiographic Evaluation of Cardiac Chambers** — 41
Global systolic function 41

Chapter 5. **Acyanotic Congenital Heart Disease** — 46
Atrial septal defect (ASD) 47
Ventricular septal defect (VSD) 51
Common atrioventricular canal 56
Patent ductus arteriosus (PDA) 58
Pulmonary stenosis (PS) 60
Congenital left ventricular outflow obstruction (LVOT) 62
Aortic stenosis 63
Coarctation of aorta 64

Chapter 6. **Cyanotic Heart Disease** — 66
Transposition of great arteries (D-TGA) 66
L-TGA 68
Tetralogy of Fallot 69

Tricuspid atresia 72
Total anomalous pulmonary venous return (TAPVR) 74
Truncus arteriosus 76

Chapter 7. **Acquired Valvular Disease** 79

Rheumatic heart disease 79
Mitral stenosis (MS) 81
Mitral regurgitation 83
Mitral valve prolapse 85
Aortic regurgitation 88
Tricuspid regurgitation 90
Tricuspid stenosis 92

Chapter 8. **Cardiac Infections** 93

Infective endocarditis 93
Pericardial disease 96

Chapter 9. **Disease of Myocardium** 101

Cardiomyopathy 101
Trauma 112

Chapter 10. **Pediatric Echocardiogram Report and its Pitfalls** 113

Errors 113

Chapter 11. **Fetal Echocardiography** 117

Indications 118
Equipment 118
Anatomic imaging 120

Chapter	12.	**Neonatal Echocardiography**	128

Persistent pulmonary hypertension (PPHN) of newborn 129
Ductal flow 129
Atrial shunting 130
Cardiac functions and output 130
Functional echocardiography 131

Chapter	13.	**Echocardiography in Intensive Care Unit**	138

Why echo in ICU? 138
Preload assessment: Prediction of volume responsiveness 138
Practical evaluation of LV systolic function 141

Index   *151*

chapter 1

Introduction

Echocardiography is a unique noninvasive method for imaging the living heart. It is based on detection of echoes produced by a beam of ultrasound (very high frequency sound) pulses transmitted into the heart.

History

Spallanzani 1700's is referred as father of ultrasound. He demonstrated that bats were blind and navigated by means of echo reflection using inaudible sound. In 1842, Christian Doppler introduced pitch of sound. Currie in 1880 discovered that first ultrasound waves were created using piezoelectrode. In 1929 Sokolov detected metal flaw, Karl Dussic in 1941, first used it in medicine. In 1950, Keidel, first used it for heart. Hertz+ and Elder in 1853, used echo for heart. In 1963, Joyner used first echo for Mitral stenosis (MS). Then in 1963, Feigenbaum placed ultrasound probe on his chest and saw moving heart images. Later in 1965, detected Feigenbaum pericardial effusion. Doppler was introduced in 1960's. Again in 1970 Color Flow was discovered. Transesophageal echo in 1982 and intracardiac Echo in 1990's were started. Hence evolved the technique of echocardiography.

It started with Motion Mode, 2-D echocrdiography and color Doppler, followed by transesophageal and intracardiac. More recently, neonatologists have become interested in the echocardiographic assessment of hemodynamic instability in infants. The terms *functional echocardiography* and *point-of-care echocardiography* have been introduced to describe the use of echocardiography as an adjunct in the clinical assessment of the hemodynamic status in neonates.[1-4] The increasing availability of echocardiography, with miniaturization of the technology, has resulted in more widespread use of echocardiography in NICUs around the world.[5] Perhaps the most significant challenge for the application of so-called functional studies is that newborns in the NICU with hemodynamic instability are at a much higher risk for having underlying congenital heart disease (CHD).

How are Echo Images Produced?

Echo images are produced by piezoelectric effect. In this electric energy is converted to crystal that makes it vibrate resulting in sound waves. The transducer frequency has characteristics of the piezocrystal. Transducer frequency is measured in MEGAHERTZ (MHz). Higher the MHz, closer is the vision.

From its introduction in 1954 to the mid 1970's, most echocardiographic studies employed a technique called M-mode, in which the ultrasound beam is aimed manually at selected cardiac structures to give a graphic recording of their positions and movements. M-mode recordings permit measurement of cardiac dimensions and detailed analysis of complex motion patterns depending on transducer angulation. They also facilitate analysis of time relationships with other physiological variables such as ECG, heart sounds, and pulse tracings, which can be recorded simultaneously.

Echocardiography animation, utilizing both M-mode and two-dimensional recordings, now 3-D and 4-D images therefore provides a great deal of information about cardiac anatomy and physiology, the clinical value of which has established echocardiography as a major diagnostic tool.

In order to understand the basic principles of echocardiography it is extremely important to understand the physical principles behind the process and also the definition of the commonly used terms.

Ultrasound is sound having frequency of > 20,000 cycles/sec. It can be directed in a beam and it obeys the laws of reflection and refraction. It is reflected by objects of small size. Ultrasound beam should be extremely narrow so that it can obtain an icepick view or slice of the heart.

Resolution is the ability to distinguish or identify two objects that are close together.

Two-dimensional (2-D) Echocardiography (Fig. 1.1) is the study of cardiac structures in a two-dimensional view.

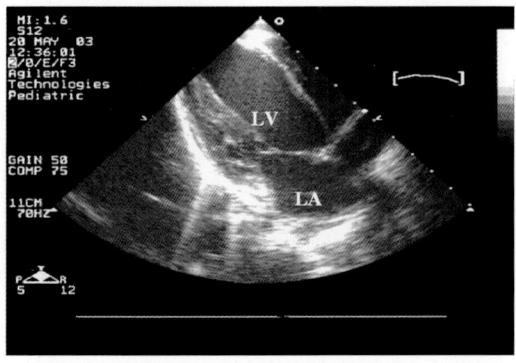

Fig. 1.1: Two-dimensional view

Three-dimensional (3-D) echo. The clinician's ability to image the heart by echocardiography had been limited to two-dimensional techniques.[6] Improving transducer technology, beam-forming and miniaturization have led to significant improvements in spatial and temporal resolution using 2-DE. However, 2-DE has fundamental limitations. The very nature of a 2-DE slice, which has no thickness, necessitates the use of multiple orthogonal 'sweeps'. The only three-dimensional image of the heart is the 'virtual image' that exists in the echocardiographer's mind, and is then translated into words. Since myocardial motion occurs in three-dimensions, 2-DE techniques inherently do not lend themselves to accurate quantitation. Early reconstructive approaches were based on 2-DE image acquisitions that were subsequently stacked and aligned based on phases of the cardiac cycle, in order to recreate a 3-DE dataset.[7–10] In 1990, von Ramm and Smith published their early results with a matrix array transducer that provided real-time images of the heart in three-dimensions.[11] Over the past five years, dramatic technological advances have facilitated the ability to perform live 3-DE scanning, including the ability to steer the beam in three-dimensions and to render the image in real time.[12] The usefulness of 3-D echocardiography has been demonstrated in (1) the evaluation of cardiac chamber volumes and mass, which avoids geometric assumptions; (2) the assessment of regional left ventricular (LV) wall motion and quantification of systolic dysynchrony; (3) presentation of realistic views of heart valves, (4) volumetric evaluation of regurgitant lesions and shunts with 3-DE color Doppler imaging, and (5) 3-DE stress imaging.

Four-dimensional (4-D) echocardiography is 3 dimensions spatial plus time.

Doppler echo is a study of cardiac structures and blood flow profiles using an ultrasound beam Doppler echocardiography is a method for detecting the direction and velocity of moving blood within the heart. Doppler examination is based on the observation that the frequency of sound increases when a source of sound is moving towards the listener and vice versa. The same applies when a reflecting object is moving towards a transducer. It is used to determine the direction and velocity of RBC with respect to ultrasound beam. The common system used is to encode flow towards the transducer as red and away from transducer as blue [BART (Blue Away; Red Toward)]. The best Doppler information is obtained when the ultrasonic beam is parallel to the moving target (opposite of that for imaging with M-mode or 2-D echo). Also better information is obtained with higher frequency transducer compared with a lower frequency transducer.

Continuous wave Doppler is used to assess valvular stenosis and regurgitation and velocity of flow inshunts.

Pulse Doppler information can be used sending a short burst of ultrasound, the frequency of that burst is distorted if the target from which it is reflected is moving. It helps to assess the normal valve functions, LV diastolic function, stroke volume and cardiac output.

The major disadvantage of the pulse Doppler system is that the velocity one can measure is limited. Pulse Doppler system has inherently pulse repetition frequency (PRF).

The PRF determines the ability of the Doppler to detect high frequency Doppler shifts. The inability of the Doppler system to detect high frequency Doppler shifts is known as aliasing. The upper limit of frequency that this limit can detect is known as *"Nyquist limit"*. This limit is one-half of PRF. If the flow exceeds this limit it is detected as flow in the opposite direction. 'Alaising' and 'wrap around' may thus add to the confusion. The Nyquist limit of color flow Doppler imaging is usually lower than ordinary pulsed spectral Doppler.

Color flow imaging is pulsed Doppler and therefore is limited in its abilities to measure high velocities. Basically two flow patterns can be detected with spectral Doppler. First is laminar, i.e. reflecting red blood cells are travelling in same direction with little difference in velocities. The Doppler signal from such a flow indicates a narrow velocity spectrum (Figs 1.2 and 1.3). Second is turbulent, this happens when blood is flowing through a narrow orifice. Multiple velocities in turbulent flows shown in Figure 1.4. As velocity increases aliasing occurs (Fig. 1.5). One of the major functions of color Doppler system is to identify abnormal flow patterns such as valvular regurgitation and shunts revealed by multiple color bands.

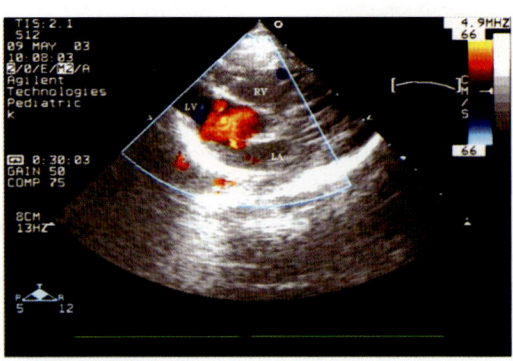

Fig. 1.2: Color flow laminar-red

Note:

- Ultrasonic beam is perpendicular to blood flow no flow or color is recorded.
- Ultrasonic beam is parallel to blood flow, e.g. apical views, high velocity, color is brighter.
- If the velocity is too low flow is not visualized.

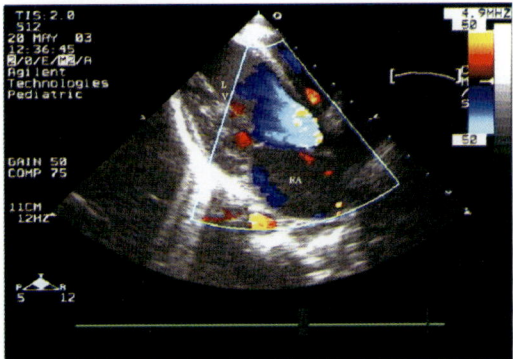

Fig. 1.3: Color flow laminar-blue

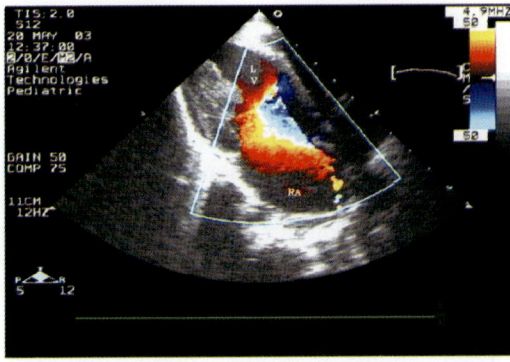

Fig. 1.4: Multiple velocities showing different colors

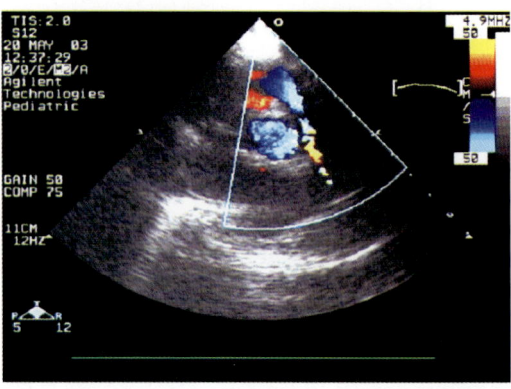

Fig. 1.5: Alaising effect

Transducers

Transthoracic

There are 4 transthoracic transducers, two phased array and two mechanical. The phased array transducers have a flat surface and no visible moving parts. The phased array transducers vary with the frequency and number of elements in the transducers. Transducers used have varying frequencies. Children frequencies vary 3.5–7.0 MHz. Higher frequency has better resolution. Adults lower frequency probe is used.

The higher frequency transducers are usually smaller. The number of elements varies from 32–128. Transducers with more elements are usually larger. The low frequency transducers have better penetration and produce better Doppler recordings. High frequency transducers give better resolution and finer image.

Transesophageal

Echo needs separate probe, adult and pediatric. Transesophageal transducers are placed in endoscopic instruments. Both mechanical and phased array devices can be used.

Intravascular

It can be placed in intravascular catheter of almost any size.

Digital Echocardiography

Digital echocardiography is the recording and display of echocardiographic data in digital form. The echocardiographic recording can be viewed and manipulated by computers.

Stress Echocardiography

Stress testing helps to identify latent or known cardiac abnormalities, only become manifest when provoked with some form of stress. Patients with valvular heart disease can show significant hemodynamic changes with stress. Doppler recordings are important under these circumstances.

Contrast Echocardiography

When liquid was injected within cardiovascular system, tiny suspended bubbles produce a cloud of echoes.

This technique is used for various purposes. The most common is right to left shunting. This technique is a sensitive means of finding small shunts.

REFERENCES

1. Kluckow AM, Seri AI, Evans AN. Functional echocardiography: An emerging clinical tool for the neonatologist. J Pediatr 2007; 150:125–30.
2. Kluckow AM, Seri AI, Evans AN. Echocardiography and the neonatologist. Pediatr Cardiol 2008; 29:1043–7.

3. Sehgal AA, McNamara APJ. Does point-of-care functional echocardiography enhance cardiovascular care in the NICU? J Perinatol 2008; 28:729–35.

4. Sehgal AA, McNamara APJ. Does echocardiography facilitate determination of hemodynamic significance attributable to the ductus arteriosus? Eur J Pediatr 2009; 168:907–14.

5. EvansAN, GournayAV, CabanasAF, KluckowAM, LeoneAT, GrovesAA, et al. Point-of-care ultrasound in the neonatal intensive care unit: International perspectives. Seminars in Fetal and Neonatal Medicine 2011; 16:61–6.

6. Tajik AJ, Seward JB, Hagler DJ, Mair DD, Lie JT. Two-dimensional real-time ultrasonic imaging of the heart and great vessels: Technique, image orientation, structure identification and validation. Mayo Clin Proc 1978; 53:271–303.

7. Ariet M, Geiser EA, Lupkiewicz SM, Conetta DA, Conti CR. Evaluation of a three-dimensional reconstruction to compute left ventricular volume and mass. Am J Cardiol1984;54:415–20.

8. Dekker DL, Piziali RL, Dong E Jr. A system for ultrasonically imaging the human heart in three-dimensions. Comput Biomed Res 1974; 7: 544–53.

9. Linker DT, Moritz WE, Pearlman AS. A new three-dimensional echocardiographic method of right ventricular volume measurement: In vitro validation. J Am Coll Cardiol 1986;8:101–6.

10. Matsumoto M, Matsuo H, Kitabatake A, Inoue M, Hamanaka Y, Tamura S, et al. Three-dimensional echocardiograms and two-dimensional echocardiographic images at desired planes by a computerized system. Ultrasound Med Biol 1977; 3: 163–78.

11. Von Ramm OT, Smith SW. Real time volumetric ultrasound imaging system. J Digital Imaging 1990; 3:261–6.

12. Salgo IS. Three-dimensional echocardiographic technology. Cardiol Clin 2007;25:231–9.

chapter 2

Position of the Patient and Transducer

Echocardiographic examination is done when the patient is flat or when he or she is in left lateral decubitus.

Windows/Views

The main echo windows are shown on the precordium (Fig. 2.1). Whether a person uses right or left hand to hold a transducer is a matter of preference. It is easier to support the transducer with four fingers rather than a thumb. The most common place to begin an examination is along left parasternal border, i.e. *left parasternal* (Fig. 2.2), the second most common location is with the transducer over the *apex* (Fig. 2.3). Both these examinations are best done with patient in left lateral decubitus. A *subcostal* approach is useful in patients who have low diaphragms and hyperinflated lungs. A subcostal view is also useful in viewing inferior vena cava and hepatic viens. The *suprasternal* (Fig. 2.4) view gives view of heart and great vessels. Both imaging and Doppler studies are performed with this examination. The subcostal (Fig. 2.5) and suprasternal studies are done with patient flat on his or her back. The *right parasternal window* helps in looking at the aorta or interatrial septum. Lesser known windows are *right apical*, *right supraclavicular fossa* and back. The right *paraspinal view* can be used for descending aorta to look for dissection.

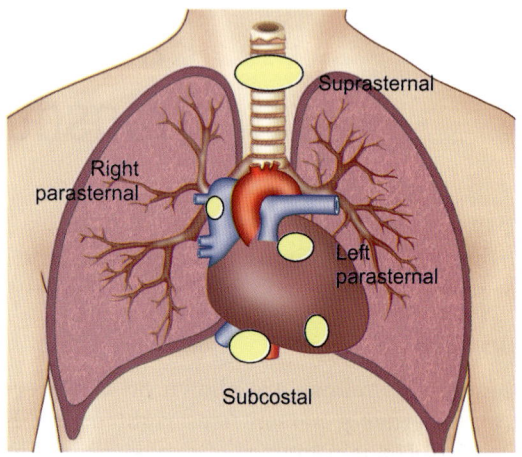

Fig. 2.1: Main echo windows

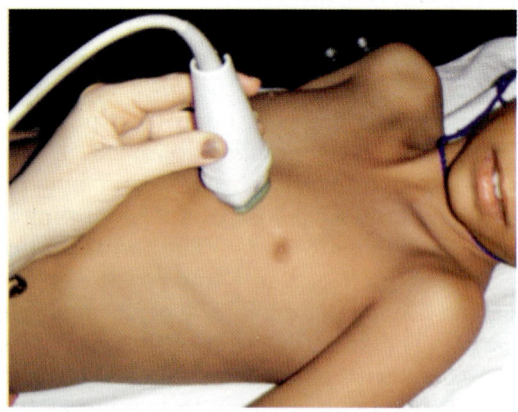

Fig. 2.2: Left parasternal view

Position of the Patient and Transducer

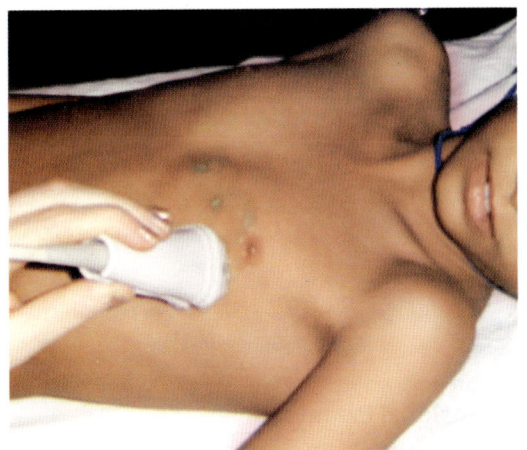

Fig. 2.3: Apical view

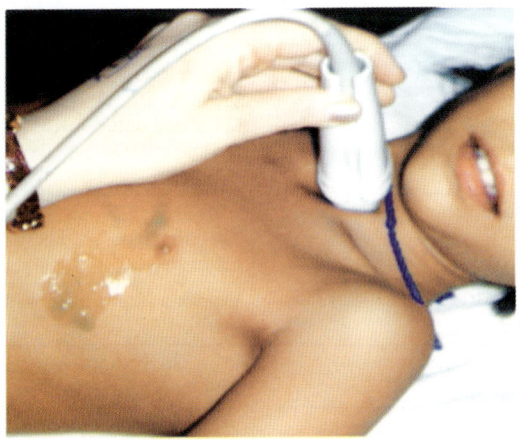

Fig. 2.4: Suprasternal view

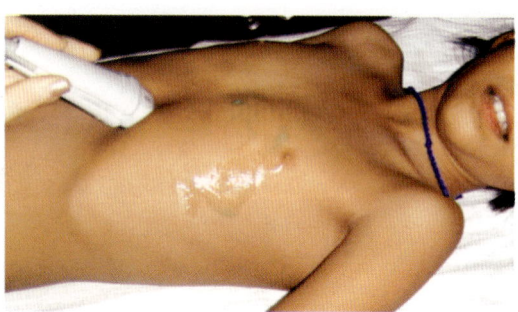

Fig. 2.5: Subcostal view

Two-Dimensional Examination

Initial approach to cardiac examination begins with two-dimensional study. The *long axis* plane runs parallel to the heart or left ventricle. The short axis is perpendicular to the long axis. The four-chamber plane is orthogonal to the other two and somewhat represents a frontal view.

Planes	Use
Parasternal long axis view (Fig. 2.6)	Visualize LV; LA; RV; LVOT; Mitral and aortic valves RV inflow TV LV apex
Parasternal short axis (Fig. 2.7)	Visualize RVOT, PV, PA branches TV, coronaries, LV, MV LV, base
Apical (four chamber view) (Fig. 2.8)	Visualize four chambers of the heart
Apical (five chamber view) (Fig. 2.9)	Visualize the aorta along the four chambers of the heart
Subcostal (Fig. 2.10)	Visualize drainage of IVC into RA
Suprasternal (Fig. 2.11)	Visualize aortic arch and its tributaries

Position of the Patient and Transducer 15

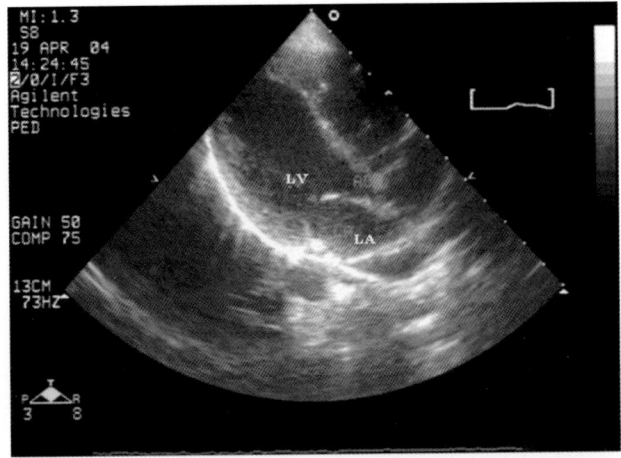

Fig. 2.6: Parasternal long axis (Plax)

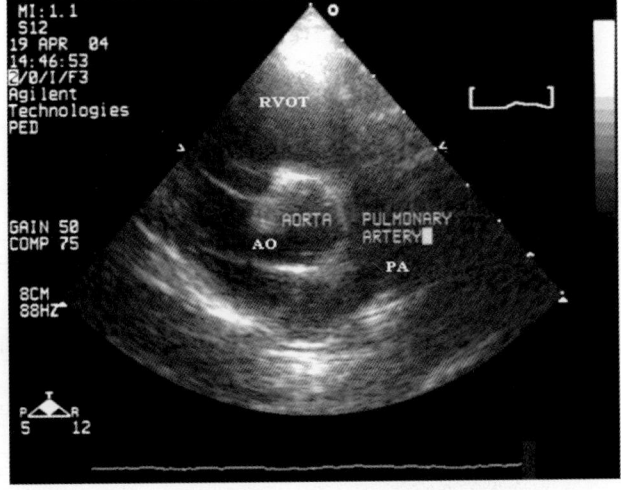

Fig. 2.7: Parasternal short axis (Psax)

16　　　　Step by Step Pediatric Echocardiography

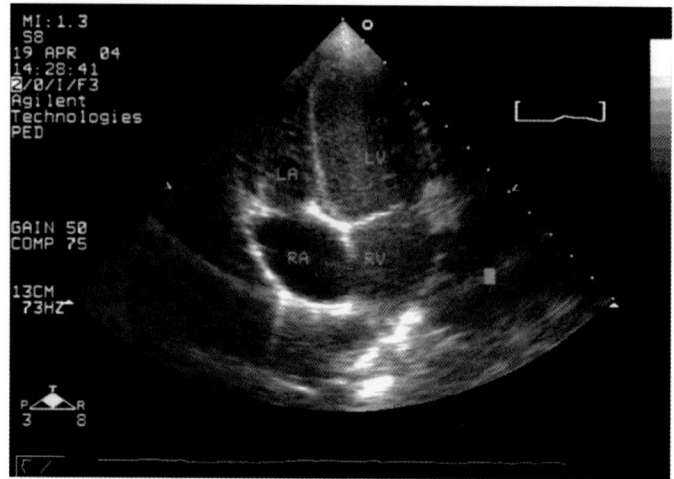

Fig. 2.8: Apical four-chamber (A 4ch)

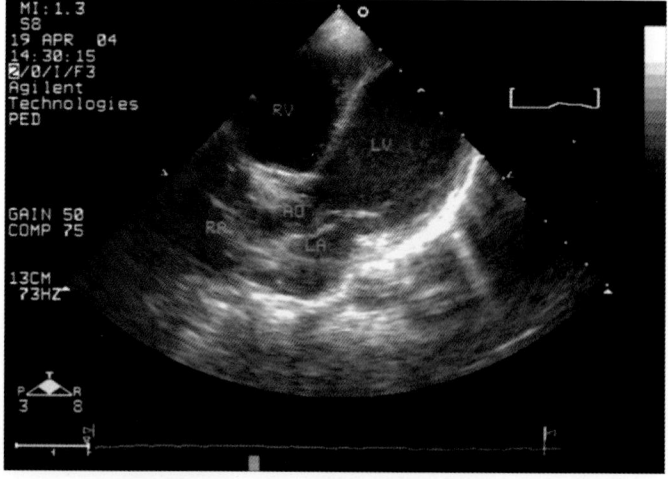

Fig. 2.9: Apical five-chamber (A 5ch)

Position of the Patient and Transducer 17

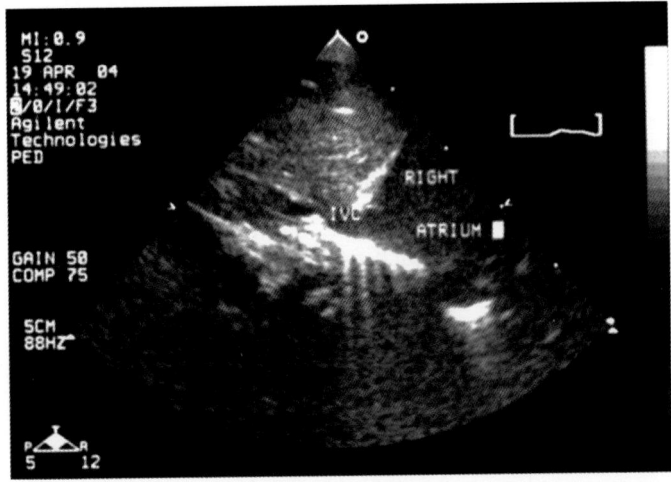

Fig. 2.10: Subxiphoid

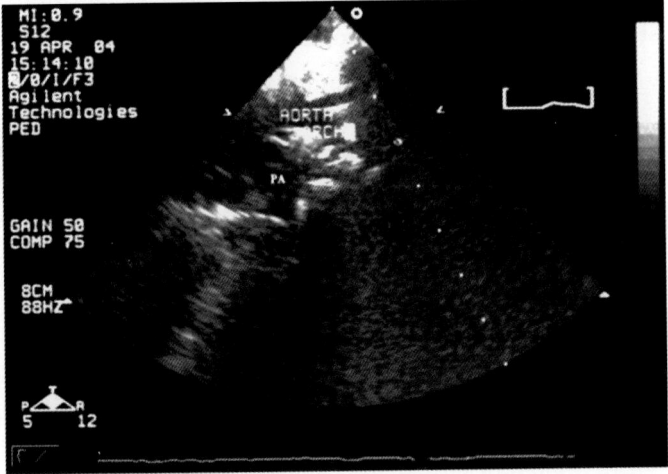

Fig. 2.11: Suprasternal aortic arch (Ach)

Normal variants

Need to be kept in mind:
- Prominent moderator band in right ventricle is frequent finding.
- Similar fine filamentous structures that traverse the left ventricular cavity represents a false chordae tendineae.
- A prominent eustachian valve is seen in the right atrium at junction of inferior vena cava and right atrium.
- Filamentous structure in right atrium represent "Chiari network". These echoes are mobile and nonpathological.
- The shape of the interventricular septum and left ventricular outflow tract may change with age. The septum becomes S-shaped or sigmoid with the arrowhead bulging into the outflow tract.

Standardized Orientation of 2-D Images

- The transducers have a index mark that indicates the edge of imaging plane, i.e. the direction in which the ultrasonic beam is swept. The index mark should be located on the transducer to indicate the edge of the image to appear on the right side of the display, e.g. parasternal long axis examination, the index mark should point in the direction of the aorta, making aorta appear on the right side of the display.
- **How is the right and left decided?**

Relative to holding the probe, there is a marker on the probe and when you hold the probe marker should point to the left. If that points to the left then you are showing left to the left of screen and right of patient to right of the screen.

Position of the Patient and Transducer 19

The different views of the heart (Figs 2.12–2.24).

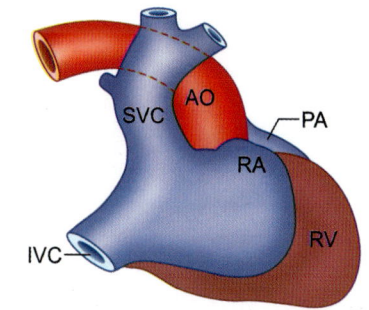

Fig. 2.12: Subxiphoid long axis (Lax)

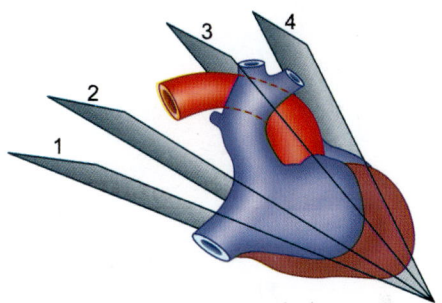

Fig. 2.13: Subxiphoid (Lax)

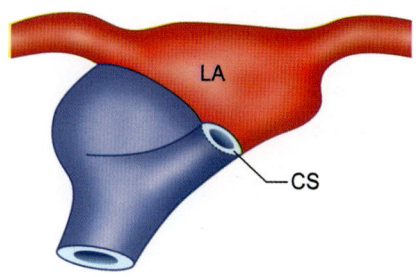

Fig. 2.14: L1

20   Step by Step Pediatric Echocardiography

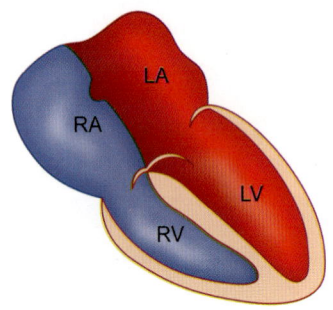

Fig. 2.15: L2

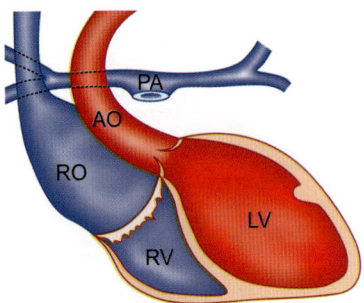

Fig. 2.16: L3

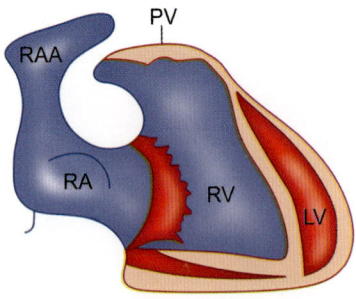

Fig. 2.17: L4

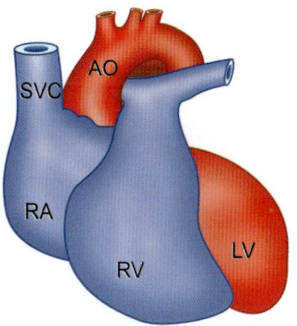

Fig. 2.18: L4

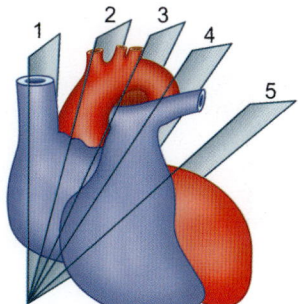

Fig. 2.19: Subxiphoid short axis

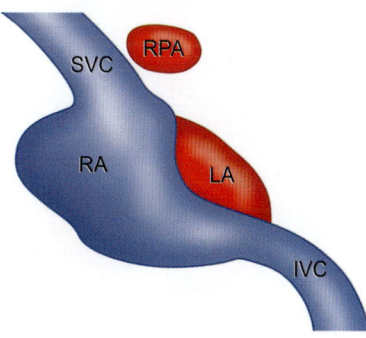

Fig. 2.20: S1

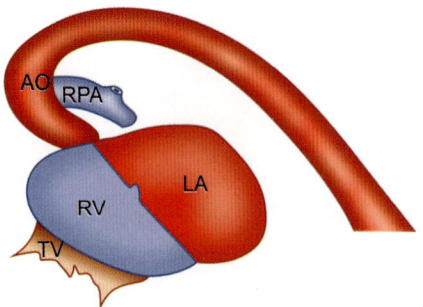

Fig. 2.21: S2

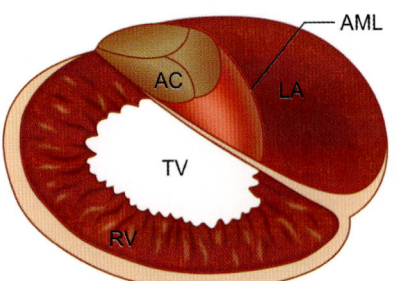

Fig. 2.22: S3

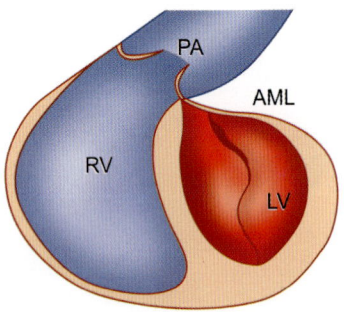

Fig. 2.23: S4

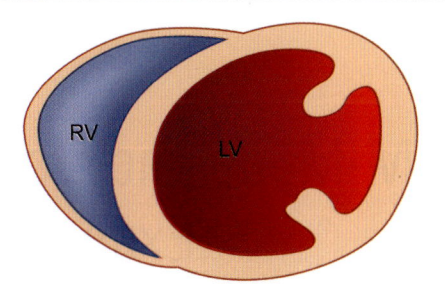

Fig. 2.24: S5

chapter

3 M-Mode and Doppler Examination

M-MODE

M-mode means the motion mode. The hallmark of M-mode echocardiography is the high temporal resolution. Distance or depth is along the vertical axis and time on the horizontal axis. The major feature is the ability to see subtle changes in wall or valve motion. Doppler examination is best done with lower frequency transducer and M-mode tracing with high frequency transducer. The beam has to be perpendicular to the cardiac walls and valve. Whereas in Doppler examination as the relationship between path of red blood cells and ultrasonic beam approaches 90, the Doppler signal drops to zero. Four view positions are described in the left parasternal view (Fig. 3.1). Most commonly used is position 2. (See Fig. 2.13).

Features of an M-mode Image

- The posterior left ventricular wall is represented by borders, the endocardial echo (EN) cavity and the epicardial echo (EP) which borders the pericardium (PER).
- The anterior mitral leaflet has an M-shaped

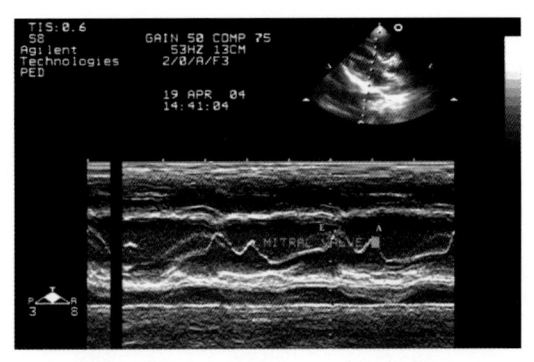

Fig. 3.1: M-mode patterns mitral valve

appearance in diastole with posterior valve leaflet assuming letter W.
- The anterior right ventricular wall is thinner than left ventricular wall and moves downward in systole and upward in diastole.
- Labelling of M-mode record of mitral valve
  - The end of systole before the opening of valve is designated as D.
  - As the anterior leaflet opens it peaks at E.
  - The peak of mitral valve motion is A. The valve begins to close with atrial relaxation.
  - Ventricular systole begins with down slope of mitral leaflet, and may produce a slight interruption in closure at B.
  - Complete closure occurs after onset of ventricular systole at C.
  - Onset of opening of mitral valve occurs at D. The PML is a mirror image of AML.

As the transducer is moved towards position (1) (See Fig. 2.13) the mitral valve is no longer visible and one may see a band of echoes originating form the

M-Mode			
Normal values	BSA(m^2)	Mean(mm)	Upper limit (mm)
LVID	0–0.5	24	32
	0.5–1.0	34	40
	>1.0	40	48
RVID	<0.50	12	18
	0.5	10	18
	>1.0	12	18
LVPW	<0.5	5	6
	0.5–1.0	6	8
	>1.0	7	8
LA	<0.5	17	24
	0.5–1.0	21	28
	1.0–1.5	24	32
Aorta	<0.5	12	16
	0.5–1.0	28	22
	>1.0	22	28

posterior papillary muscle. The posterior left ventricular wall becomes the left atrial wall (PLA). The PLA is characterized by the lack of systolic anterior motion. The wall is thinner and the motion is primarily in diastole. Moving the cursor to position (4) (See Fig. 2.13) aortic valve, aorta and left atrium become visible (Fig. 3.2).

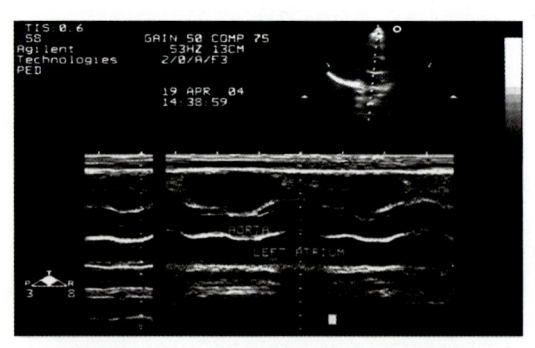

Fig. 3.2: M-mode patterns aortic root and LA

Doppler velocity values in children

Velocities	Range	Mean
Tricuspid valve	0.3–0.8 m/sec	0.6
Mitral valve	0.8–1.3 m/sec	1.0
Aortic valve	1.0–1.8 m/sec	1.5
Pulmonic valve	0.7–1.2 m/sec	1.0

Doppler gradient

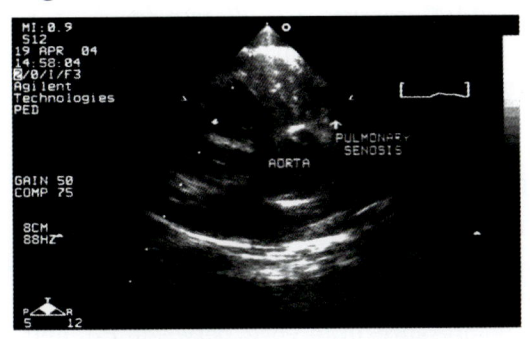

Fig. 3.3: Pulmonary valvular stenosis

Valvular stenosis (Fig. 3.3)

PS/AS/Coarctation of aorta can be assessed by Doppler gradient across valve or obstruction.

- PS/AS Severity—Assessment
  - Gradient >15 mmHg—Abnormal
  - Upto 50 mmHg—Mild
  - 50– 75 mmHg—Moderate
  - > 75 mmHg—Severe.
- Coarctation gradient >30 mmHg—Significant.

Mitral Valve-Tricuspid Valve

It is assessed by measuring:
- Valve gradient (peak; mean)

- Valve area indirectly (pressure half time)
  - MS: Normal MVA—4–6 cm^2/m^2
  - Mild MS-Above—1.5 cm^2/m^2
  - Moderate MS—1–1.5 cm^2/m^2
  - Severe MS—<1 cm^2/m^2
  - TS—Severe TS <1.3 cm^2.
- Right arm systolic BP – Interventricular (IV) gradient = RVSP = PA pressure
- Normal PA pressure = 25–30 mmHg
  - Mild PAH 30–50 mmHg
  - Moderate PAH 50–75 mmHg
  - Severe PAH > 75 mmHg.

Tricuspid Regurgitation (Fig. 3.4)

- Peak gradient +10 mmHg = RVSP (Fig. 3.5).
- PR gives PA diastolic pressure.
- Trivial PR is physiological.
- PR is pressure difference between PA and RV in diastole.

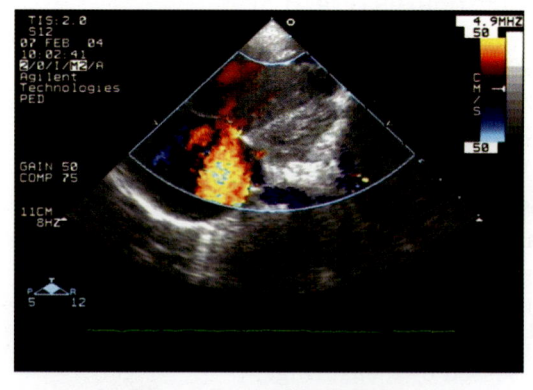

Fig. 3.4: Tricuspid regurgitation

- RVEDP + PR jet = PA diastolic pressure.
- Normal PA diastolic pressure is 10–15 mmHg.

DOPPLER ECHOCARDIOGRAPHY

It is described by Austrian Physicist Christian Johann Doppler in 1842. It's a change in the frequency of sound, light or other waves caused by motion of the source. Ultrasound waves of known frequency are transmitted from the transducer and are reflected by moving blood back towards the ultrasound receiver. If the blood is moving towards the transducer the frequency increases and vice versa. This is then used by the computer analysis to derive hemodynamic information. The Doppler measured flow patterns and velocities across the valves can be displayed graphically against time on screen of the machine. By convention the velocities towards the transducer are displayed above the baseline and those away from the transducer below the line.

It is the method of detecting the direction and velocity of moving blood within the heart and great vessels. Also used to detect valve stenosis, regurgitation, flow across a shunt, etc. evaluating normal and abnormal flow states. (Fig. 3.6).

It works on the principle that laminar flow in the cardiac chamber and vessels (Fig. 3.6). Turbulent flow is present when there is some obstruction disrupting normal laminar flow pattern. Causing the orderly movement of RBCs to become disorganized and produce various whirls and eddies of differing velocities and directions. Obstruction to the flow also results in increase in velocity. Echo emits high frequency burst of sound(ultrasound) into the tissue.

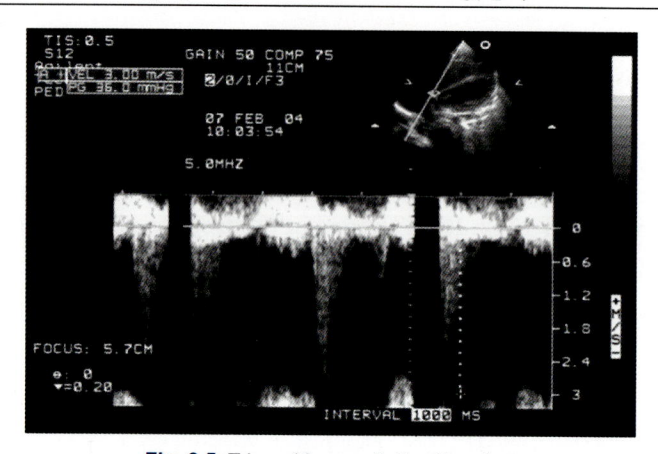

Fig. 3.5: Tricuspid regurgitation Dopplers

Laminar flow

Turbulent flow

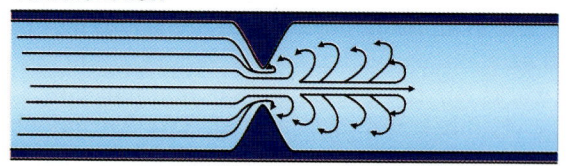

Fig. 3.6: Laminar and turbulent flow

Frequency

Frequency is a fundamental characteristics of any wave phenomenon and refers to the number of waves that pass a given point in one second (Fig. 3.7).

Described in units of cycles per second or Hertz(Hz).

Doppler echocardiography depends entirely on measurement of the relative change in the returned ultrasound frequency when compared to the transmitted frequency and measures the direction, velocity and turbulance of disturbed flow (Fig. 3.7).

Doppler shift = 2fo/c.VCosθ(Fig. 3.8)
fo = transmitted frequency (Fig. 3.9)
V = velocity of the moving blood (Fig. 3.10)
c = constant, velocity of sound in blood.

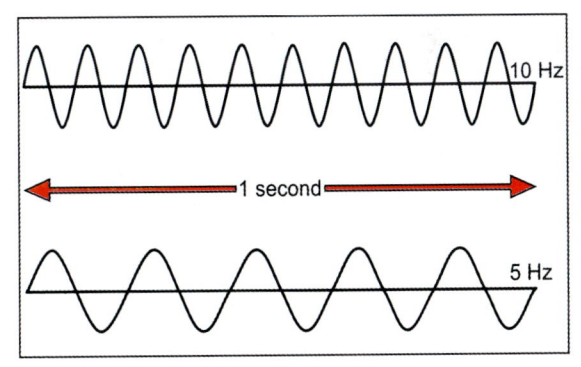

Fig. 3.7: Frequency

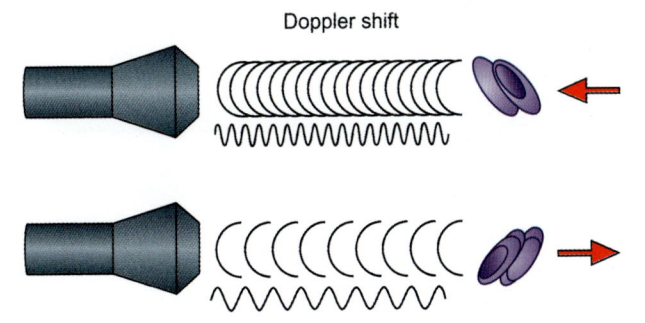

Fig. 3.8: Doppler shift

$$F_o = \frac{2t_o}{C} V \cos\theta$$

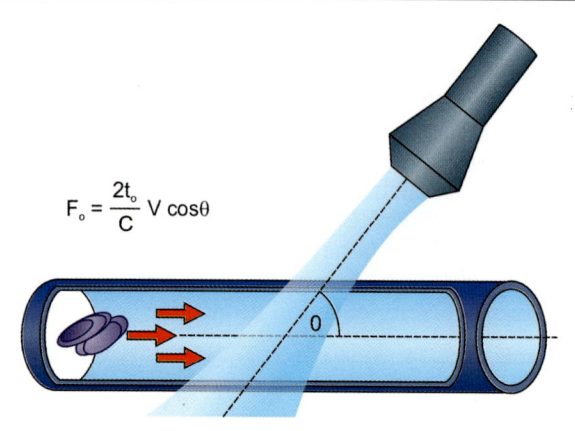

Fig. 3.9: Transmitted frequency

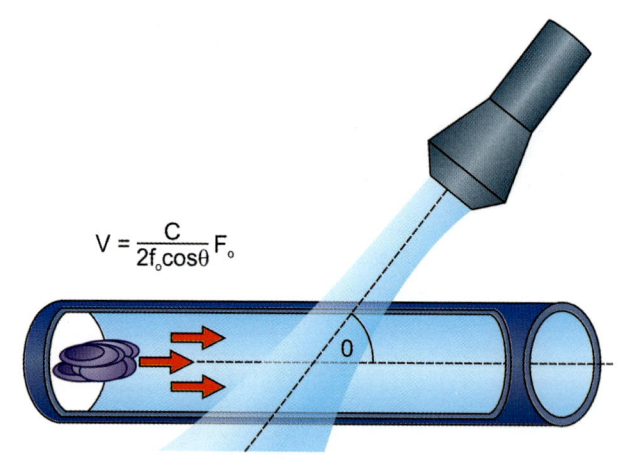

$$V = \frac{C}{2f_o \cos\theta} F_o$$

Fig. 3.10: Velocity of blood

Flow velocity toward the transducer is displayed as a positive or upward shift in velocity (Fig. 3.11). Flow velocity away from the transducer is displayed as a negative or downward shift. Time is on the horizontal axis.

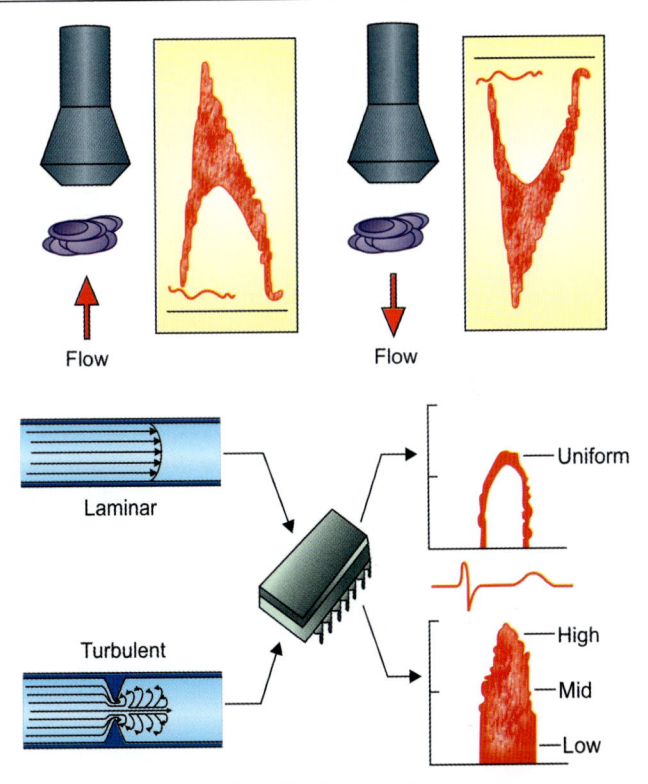

Fig. 3.11: Flow velocity

Pulsed and Continuous Wave Doppler

There are two main types of Doppler echocardiographic systems in common use today, continuous wave and pulsed wave. They differ in transducer design and operating features, signal processing procedures and in the types of information provided. Each has important advantages and disadvantages and, in our opinion, the current practice of Doppler echocardiography requires some capability for both forms.

Continuous Wave Doppler

Continuous wave (CW) Doppler is the older and electronically more simple of the two kinds. As the name implies, CW Doppler involves continuous generation of ultrasound waves coupled with continuous ultrasound reception. A two crystal transducer accomplishes this dual function with one crystal devoted to each function (Fig. 3.12).

The main advantage of CW Doppler is its ability to measure high blood velocities accurately. Indeed, CW Doppler can accurately record the highest velocities in any valvular and congenital heart disease. Since velocities exceeding 1.5 m/sec are frequently seen in such disorders, accurate high velocity measurement is of particular importance for allowing the recognition of the full abnormal flow profile. It is also of considerable importance for the quantitative evaluation of abnormal flows, as will be seen later.

The main disadvantage of CW Doppler is its lack of

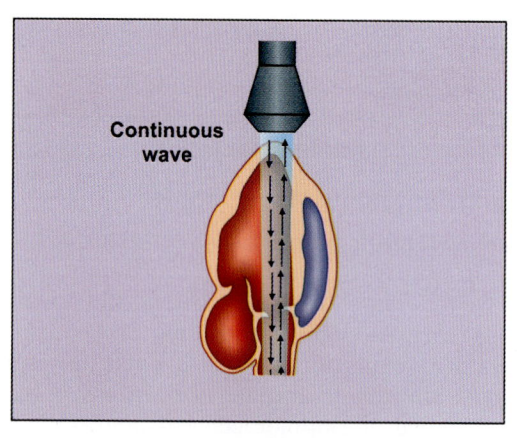

Fig. 3.12: Two crystal transducer for CW

selectivity or depth discrimination. Since CW Doppler is constantly transmitting and receiving from two different transducer heads (crystals) there is no provision for imaging or range gating to allow selective placing of a given Doppler sample volume in space. As a consequence, the output from a CW examination contains Doppler shift data from every red cell reflecting ultrasound back to the transducer along the course of the ultrasound beam.

Thus, true CW Doppler is functionally a stand-alone technique whether or not the capability is housed within a two-dimensional imaging transducer. The absence of anatomic information during CW examination may lead to interpretive difficulties, particularly if more than one heart chamber or blood vessel lies in the path of the ultrasound beam.

It is possible, however, to program a phased array system to perform both two-dimensional and CW Doppler functions almost simultaneously. The quasisimultaneous CW-imaging uses a time sharing arrangement in which the transducer rapidly switches

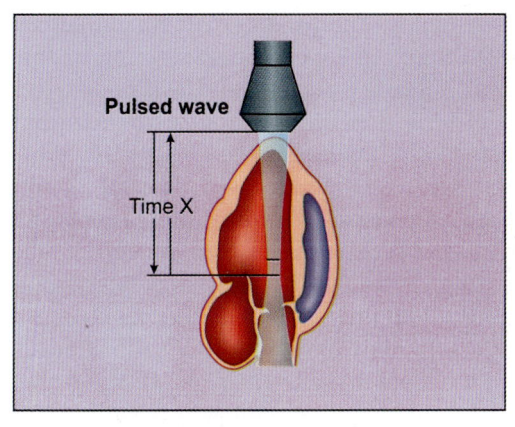

Fig.3.13: Pulsed wave Doppler

back and forth from one type of examination to the other. Because this switching is done at very high speeds, the operator gets the impression that both studies are being done continuously and in real-time. During the imaging period, no Doppler data is being collected, so an estimate is generated, usually from the preceding data. During the Doppler collection period, previously stored image data is displayed. This arrangement usually degrades the quality of both the image and Doppler data.

Pulsed wave (PW) Doppler systems use a transducer that alternates transmission and reception of ultrasound in a way similar to the M-mode transducer (Fig. 3.13). One main advantage of pulsed Doppler is its ability to provide Doppler shift data selectively from a small segment along the ultrasound beam, referred to as the "sample volume". The location of the sample volume is operator controlled. An ultrasound pulse is transmitted into the tissues travels for a given time (time X) until it is reflected back by a moving red cell. It then returns to the transducer over the same time interval but at a shifted frequency. The total transit time to and from the area is 2X. Since the speed of ultrasound in the tissues is constant, there is a simple relationship between round trip travel time and the location of the sample volume relative to the transducer face (i.e. distance to sample volume equals ultrasound speed divided by round trip travel time). This process is alternately repeated through many transmit-receive cycles each second.

This range gating is therefore dependent on a timing mechanism that only samples the returning Doppler shift data from a given region. It is calibrated so that as the operator chooses a particular location for the sample volume, the range gate circuit will permit only Doppler shift data from inside that area to be displayed as output.

All other returning ultrasound information is essentially "ignored".

Another main advantage of PW Doppler is the fact that some imaging may be carried on alternately with the Doppler and thus the sample volume may be shown on the actual two-dimensional display for guidance. PW Doppler capability is possible in combination with imaging from a mechanical or phased array imaging system. It is also generally steerable through the two-dimensional field of view, although not all systems have this capability.

In reality, since the speed of sound in body tissues is constant, it is not possible to simultaneously carry on both imaging and Doppler functions at full capability in the same ultrasound system. In mechanical systems, the cursor and sample volume are positioned during real-time imaging, and the two-dimensional image is then frozen when the Doppler is activated. With most phased array imaging systems the Doppler is variably programed to allow periodic update of a single frame

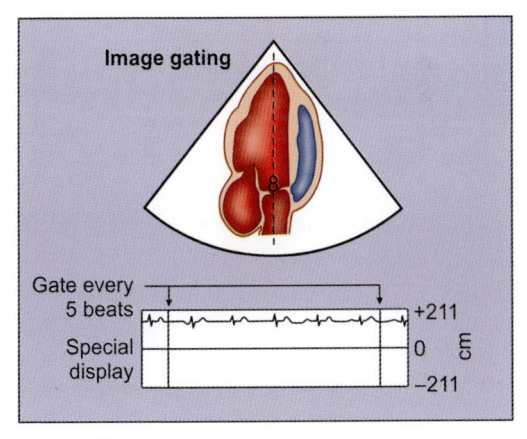

Fig.3.14: 2-D images every few beats

two-dimensional image every few beats (Fig. 3.14). In other phased arrays, two-dimensional frame rate and line density are significantly decreased to allow enough time for the PW Doppler to sample effectively. This latter arrangement gives the appearance of near simultaneity.

The sample volume is really a three-dimensional, teardrop-shaped portion of the ultrasound beam (Fig. 3.15). Its volume varies with different Doppler machines, different size and frequency transducers and different depths into the tissue. Its width is determined by the width of the ultrasound beam at the selected depth. Its length is determined by the length of each transmitted ultrasound pulse.

Therefore, the farther into the heart the sample volume is moved, the larger it effectively becomes. This happens because the ultrasound beam diverges as it gets farther away from the transducer.

The main disadvantage of PW Doppler is its inability to accurately measure high blood flow velocities, such as may be encountered in certain types of valvular and

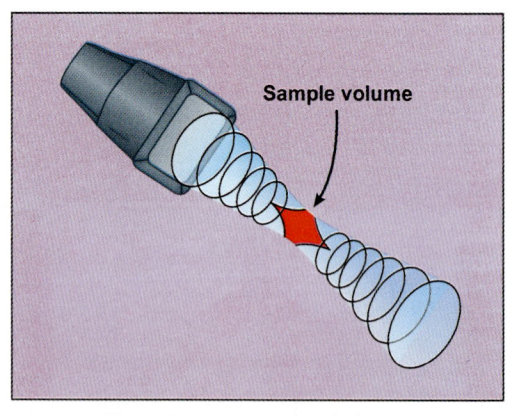

Fig.3.15: Sample volume teardrop

congenital heart disease. This limitation is technically known as "aliasing" and results in an inability of pulsed Doppler to faithfully record velocities above 1.5–2 m/sec when the sample volume is located at standard ranges in the heart (Fig. 3.16). Aliasing is represented on the spectral trace as a cut-off of a given velocity with placement of the cut section in the opposite channel or reverse flow direction. Because aliasing is so common in disease states, it will be considered in more detail in the next section.

The spectral outputs from PW and CW appear differently (Fig. 3.17). When there is no turbulence, PW will generally show a laminar (narrow band) spectral output. CW, on the other hand, rarely displays such a neat narrow band of flow velocities even with laminar flow because all the various velocities encountered by the ultrasound beams are detected by CW.

It can usually be said that when an operator wants to know where a specific area of abnormal flow is located

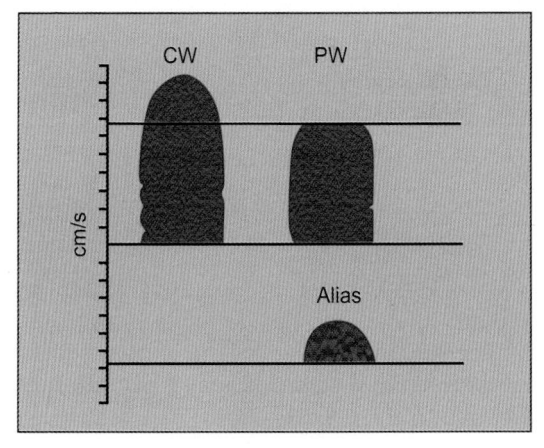

Fig. 3.16: Aliasing

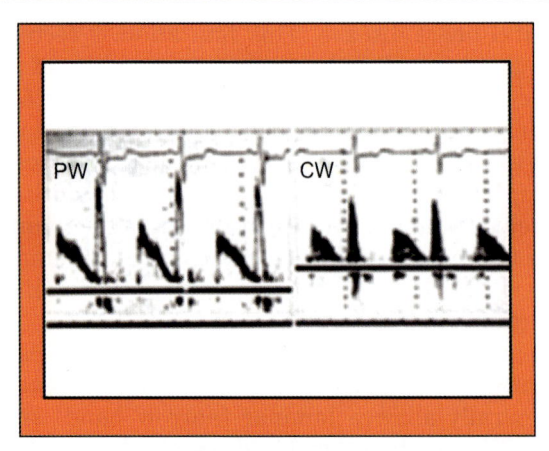

Fig.3.17: Spectral outputs of PW and CW

Comparison of pulsed and continuous wave techniques

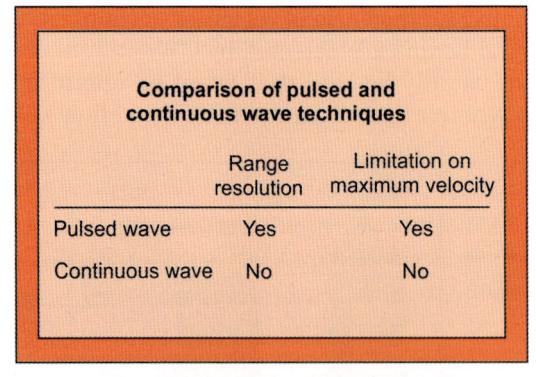

	Range resolution	Limitation on maximum velocity
Pulsed wave	Yes	Yes
Continuous wave	No	No

Fig.3.18: Comparison of PW and CW

that pulsed wave Doppler is indicated. When accurate measurement of elevated flow velocity is required, then CW Doppler should be used. The various differences between pulsed and continuous wave Doppler are summarized in Figure 3.18.

chapter 4
Echocardiographic Evaluation of Cardiac Chambers

GLOBAL SYSTOLIC FUNCTION

Left Ventricle

Ejection fraction represents the percent or fraction of left ventricular diastolic volume which is ejected in systole (stroke volume/diastolic volume). Some authors report that one can make a reasonable "eyeball" estimate of ejection fraction from 2-D echo, without actual measurements.

A simple echocardiographic measurement for assessing global systolic function is the mitral E point septal separation. This measurement is usually obtained from M-mode echocardiogram (normal distance from E point to left side of septum < 1 cm). As the left ventricle dilates the septum moves anteriorly, also a decrease in amplitude of mitral valve E point reflects a poorer flow through the valve or poor stroke volume. Hence, there is an increase in distance, between the mitral valve E point and interventricular septum with decreased ejection fraction.

Common measurements

- Ejection fraction 66±4%
- Fraction shortening 36±4%.

Diastolic function

Spectral Doppler is currently the recommended technique for evaluation.

LV diastolic dysfunction produces two patterns of flow.

- *Reduced height of E wave and increased height of A wave-associated with prolonged isovolumetric relaxation time(IVVR) and slower fall in pressure as seen in*:
  - Left ventricular hypertrophy
  - Myocardial ischemia
  - Cardiomyopathy
  - Aging
  - Filling pressure is low as in dehydration or hypovolemia
  - Flow to left side is reduced because of PAH.
- *Reverse pattern (E wave may be taller and A wave shorter): Left atrial pressure is high leading to short IVVR.*
  - Mitral regurgitation
  - Congestive heart failure
  - Restrictive CMP.

Wall thickness (Figs 4.1A and B)

M-mode can be used to measure thickness of interventricular septum (SWT) and posterior left ventricular wall (LVWT). 2-D echo can also be used to measure the wall thickness.

Right Ventricle

The echocardiographic examination of right ventricle has many difficulties, since RV lies beneath the sternum,

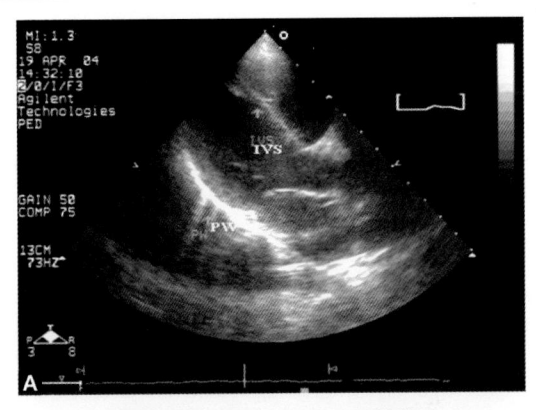

Fig. 4.1A: Measurement of SWT

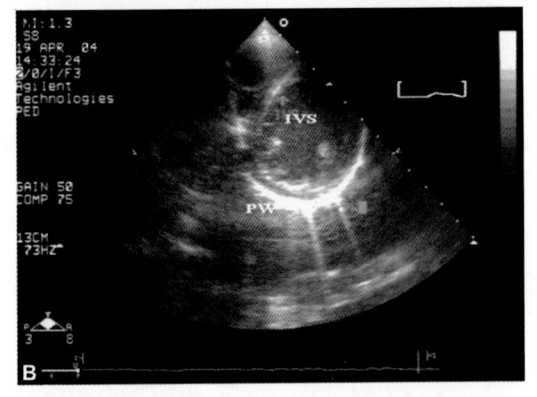

Fig. 4.1B: Measurement of LVWT

chamber is irregular in shape, the walls are trabeculated and its location within the chest is variable with the position of the patient.

Right ventricle dimension, area and volume is assessed on apical four chamber view. If right ventricular area equals or exceeds left ventricular area, one can assume, that it is dilated. No accepted technique is used for calculating right ventricular volumes or global systolic function because measurement of right ventricle is difficult to obtain. Right ventricle pressure overload is detected by pressure hypertrophy of right ventricle. Dilatation of right ventricle is an indicator of volume overload.

Left Atrium (Fig. 4.2)

Qualitative assessment of left atrial size is done by comparing the left atrial dimension to diameter of aorta. In normal subjects, the diameter of aorta and that of left atrium are equal. As LA dilates this relationship changes. Another useful sign of LA dilatation is bulging of interatrial septum towards right atrium. This is noted in four chamber view. One can see definite flow in atrial appendage when patient is in sinus rhythm; however with atrial flutter or fibrillation, a marked change in flow pattern is evident within atrial appendage. The left atrium, specially the atrial appendage is a common site for thrombosis.

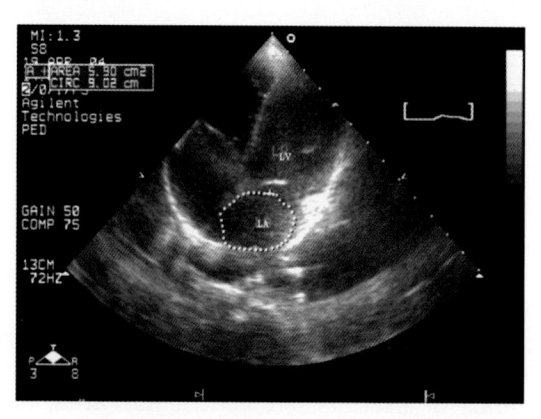

Fig. 4.2: Measurement of area and length of LA

Right Atrium

The best site to visualize it is the four chamber view. The shape of interatrial septum, and comparison with left atrium helps to assess its size.

chapter 5

Acyanotic Congenital Heart Disease

2-D echocardiography has played a phenomenal role in diagnosis of congenital heart disease, and Doppler, its correct hemodynamic status.

Segmental Approach to CHD

- Identify morphologically each cardiac segment independently, i.e. atria, ventricles, and great vessels.
- Their connections and relations are defined.

Cardiac Situs

Atrial situs solitus is the normal situation, best studied in the subcostal view, morphologic right atrium to the right, and the left atrium to the left. Atrial and visceral situs are almost always concordant. Pulmonary venous connection is seen in four chamber and suprasternal view.

Atrial Situs

- Visceral situs (visceroatrial concordance)
- Atrial morphology (situs solitus or inversus)
- Venous inflow patterns
- Ventricular loop, D loop or L loop
- AV concordance.

Identification of Cardiac Chambers	
Right	**Left**
Atria	
Eustachian valve present	Absent
Appendage short and broad	Long, thin, and narrow
Elongated shape	Rounded
Ventricles	
Trabeculated endocardial surface	Smooth endocardial surface
Chordae insert into ventricular septum	Two papillary muscle
Triangular cavity	Ellipsoidal geometry
TV with relatively apical insertion	MV with relatively basal insertion

The four-chamber view helps to determine ventricular morphology and relative position of atrioventricular valves.

Great Artery Connections

Identification of great arteries is the final step in segmental approach to cardiac anatomy. The morphologic left ventricle gives rise to aorta, and pulmonary artery outlet of right ventricle. In L-Transposition atrioventricular discordance is present, so the morphological right ventricle lies to the left of morphologic left ventricle.

ATRIAL SEPTAL DEFECT (ASD)

- Isolated anomaly in 5–10% M:F:;1:2
- 30–50% of children have ASD as part of cardiac defects.

Pathology

Three types—Secundum, primum, and sinus venosus.

The PFO does not ordinarily produce intracardiac shunts.

Ostium secundum (Fig. 5.1) is the most common type of ASD (50–70%). The defect is present in fossa ovalis, allowing shunting of blood from LA to RA.

Ostium primum occurs in 30% of all ASDs including those as a part of complete atrioventricular defects. Isolated ostium ASD occurs in 15% of all ASD.

Sinus venosus occurs in 10% of all defects. It is commonly located at the entry of SVC into RA and rarely at the entry of IVC into the RA.

Clinical Manifestations

- Children and infants usually asymptomatic.
- A widely split S2 and a grade 2-3/6 ejection systolic murmur are characteristic.
- Large shunts have a mid diastolic rumble due to relative TS audible at LLSB.
- Typical findings may be absent in children with large defects.

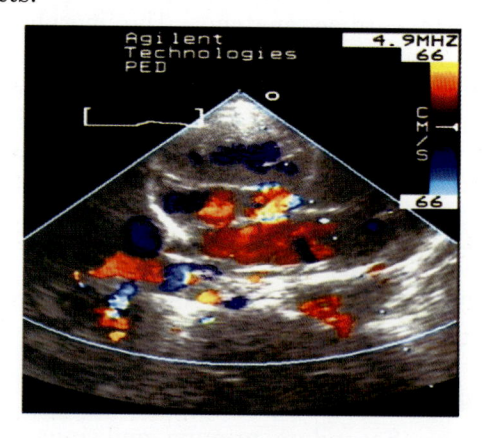

Fig. 5.1: ASD secundum

ECG

RAD of +90 to +180 degrees and mid RVH or RBBB with an rsR' pattern in V1.

X-ray chest

- Cardiomegaly with RA and RV enlargement is visible.
- A prominent MPA segment and increased PVMs can be seen.

Echocardiography

- 2-D echo is diagnostic. It shows position as well as the size of the defect.
- Indirect signs of left to right shunt.
  - RVE and RAE and dilated PA.
  - Pulse Doppler: Characteristic flow pattern with maximum left to right shunt during diastole.
  - Doppler estimates pressures in RV and PA.
  - M-mode - increased RV size and paradoxical motion of IVS - signals of RV volume overload.

Natural History

Spontaneous closure of secundum defect occurs in first 4 years of life.

Most children remain asymptomatic though CHF may rarely occur in infancy. With or without surgery atrial flutter or fibrillation occurs in adults.

Infective endocarditis does not occur with isolated ASD.

Patent Foramen Ovale (Fig. 5.2)

There is discontinuity between upper margin of septum primum and limbus of the foramen ovale, the septum primum is redundant not deficient as seen in secundum.

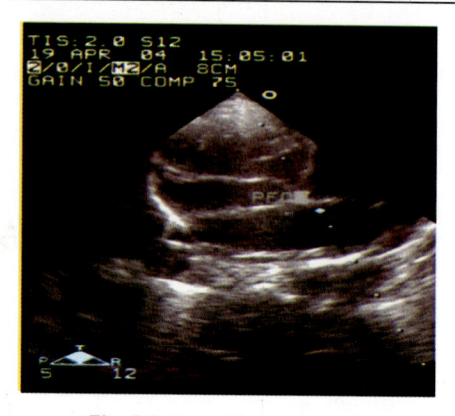

Fig. 5.2: Patent foramen ovale

Views

- Subxyphoid L2 and S2
- Right sternal border.

Ostium Primum (Fig. 5.3)

Deficiency of the lower atrial septum above the atrioventricular valves.

Views

- Subxiphoid L2-3, and S2-3

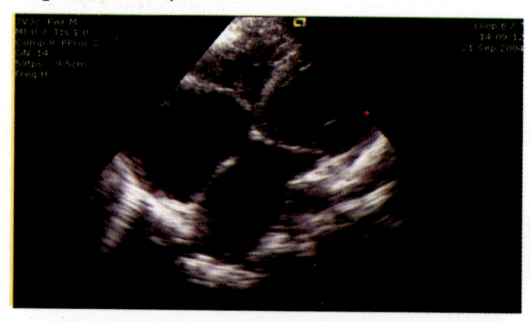

Fig. 5.3: Ostium primum

- Apical four-chambered view
- Precordial short axis view.

Problems

- Dilated coronary sinus may give false impression.
- Commonly associated lesions with ASD primum are:
  - Inlet VSD.
  - Cleft mitral valve.
  - Presence and severity of atrioventricular valve regurgitation.
  - Partial attachment of septal leaflet of mitral valve to IV septum.

Atrial Septal Defect (Sinus Venosus) (Fig. 5.4)

It occurs in 10% of all ASDs, most commonly located at entry of SVC into RA and rarely at entry of IVC into RA.

VENTRICULAR SEPTAL DEFECT (VSD)

Most common form of CHD and accounting for 15–20% of CHDs.

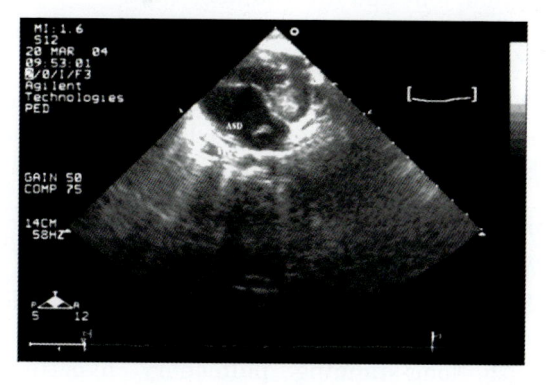

Fig. 5.4: ASD sinus venosus

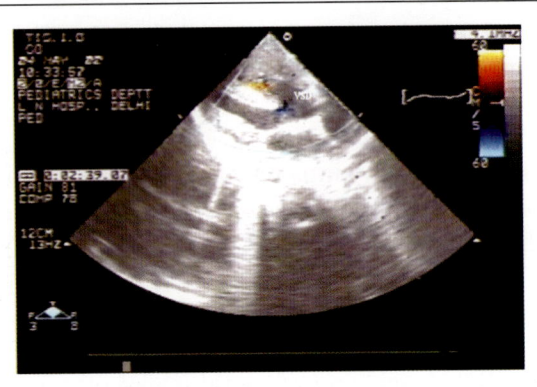

Fig. 5.5: Ventricular septal defect

Views for VSD Evaluation

- Membranous (Fig. 5.5)
  - Apical— Just under the aortic valve
  - Parasternal (SA) at level of AV, adjacent to TV.
- Muscular
  - Inlet— Apical view beneath AV valves.
  - Trabecular—Parasternal (LA) central, apical, marginal, four and five chamber view.
  - Outlet/infundibular (beneath aortic valve, e.g. TOF) - parasternal (LA).

The defect varies from small, (Fig. 5.6) having no hemodynamic consequence, to large defect leading to CHF and pulmonary hypertension.

Clinical Presentations

- With small VSD, patient is asymptomatic.
- With large VSD, delayed growth and development, repeated pulmonary infections and CHF.
- With long-standing pulmonary hypertension, a history of cyanosis and a decreased activity.

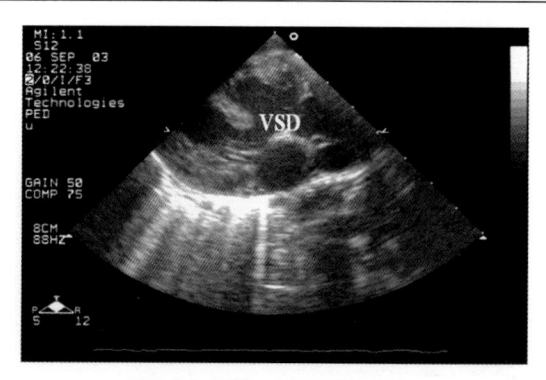

Fig. 5.6: VSD perimembranous

ECG

- Small VSD, ECG is normal.
- With moderate VSD, LVH and occasional LAH may be seen.
- Large defect, ECG shows combined ventricular hypertrophy (CVH).
- If PVOD develops, ECG shows RVH only.

X-ray

Cardiomegaly (LA, LV and RV increase). MPA and hilar PA enlarge in PVOD.

Echocardiography

- Confirm (VSD).
- Determine size and site of VSD and turbulence on color flow (Fig. 5.7).
- Rule out associated lesions like aortic regurgitation (Fig. 5.8).
- Estimate right ventricular and pulmonary arterial pressure.
- In a large shunt there may be enlargement of LV, RV, LA.

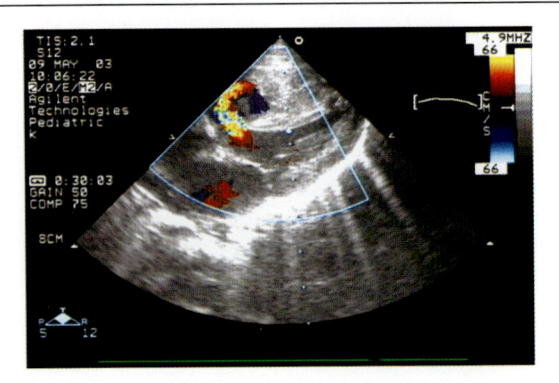

Fig. 5.7: VSD-color flow

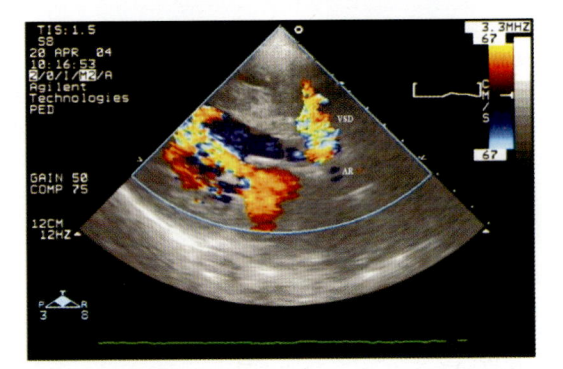

Fig. 5.8: VSD with aortic regurgitation

- Interventricular gradient (Fig. 5.9)
  - Doppler cursor in the RV side of VSD will give a positive jet from the baseline in left to right shunt (Fig. 5.10).
  - Right arm systolic BP – IV gradient = RVSP = PA pressure.
  - Normal PA pressure—25–30 mmHg
    - Mild PAH— 30–50 mmHg

Acyanotic Congenital Heart Disease 55

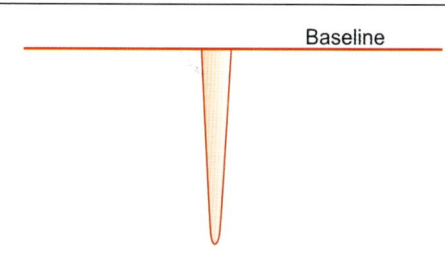

Fig. 5.9: Interventricular gradient

- Moderate PAH— 50– 75 mmHg
- Severe—PAH > 75 mmHg.
- Criteria for diagnosis
  - These defects may be seen as drop out echoes from interventricular septum, to be more definitive, they are seen in more than one view.
  - Additional findings
    - Left atrial enlargement
    - Left ventricular enlargement
    - Doppler reveals turbulence at right septal margin.

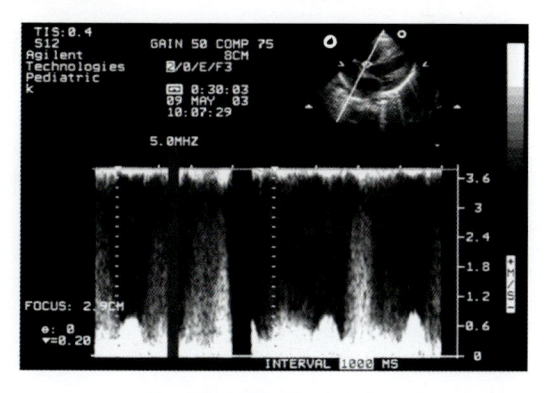

Fig. 5.10: VSD Doppler flow

Complications Associated with VSD

- Ventricular septal aneurysm.
- Aortic regurgitation (common with outlet defects) [Implication – surgical closure is indicated in absence of large shunt to reduce risk of progressive AV dysfunction].
- Vegetation on RV side.

Natural History

- Spontaneous closure in 30–40% with membranous and muscular VSD in first 6 months.
- CHF develops in infants with large VSD not before 4–8 weeks.
- PVOD develops as early as 6–12 months. with large VSD but R–L shunts not till teenage.

COMMON ATRIOVENTRICULAR CANAL (FIG. 5.11)

2% of all CHDs. Of the patients with common AV canal 30% are of Down's syndrome.

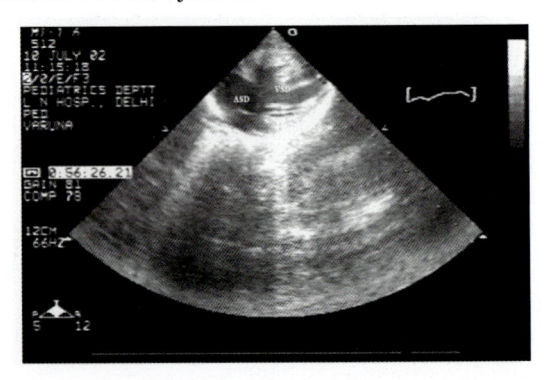

Fig. 5.11: Common AV canal

Pathology

Common AV canal usually involves structures derived from endocardial cushion tissue. Ostium primum, ASD, VSD in inlet ventricular septum, cleft in anterior mitral valve and septal leaflet of tricuspid valve is affected in complete ECD.

When two AV valves are present without interventricular shunt, the defect is ostium primum ASD.

Clinical Manifestation

Failure to thrive, recurrent respiratory infections and signs of CHF are the usual presenting features.

ECG

Prolonged PR interval. RVH, or RBBB are present in all cases and some have LVH too.

X-ray chest

Cardiomegaly, involving all four chambers.

Echocardiography

- 2-D and Doppler echo allow imaging of:
  - Size of ASD
  - Size of VSD
  - Size of AV valves
  - Anatomy of leaflets
  - Chordal attachment
  - Absolute size of RV and LV
  - AV valve regurgitation.
- Views
  - Precordial short axis
  - Apical four chamber views
  - Subxiphoid L2– 3, S3 – 4.

- Diagnostic criteria
  - There is atrioventricular canal type VSD with divided A-V valve crossing interventricular septum. ASD primum.

Natural History of AV Canal Defect

- CHF in 1–2 months and recurrent pneumonia.
- Without surgical intervention most patients die by 2–3 years of age.
- In later half of first year, they develop PVOD.

PATENT DUCTUS ARTERIOSUS (PDA)

PDA occurs in 5–10% of all CHDs, excluding preterm patients. M:F::1:3.

Pathology

- Pulmonary arterial end of the ductus is to the left of pulmonary trunk and adjacent to LPA (Fig. 5.12). Aortic insertion is opposite and just beyond origin of subclavian artery.
- The ductus is usually cone-shaped with a small orifice to the PA, which is restrictive to blood flow (Fig. 5.13).

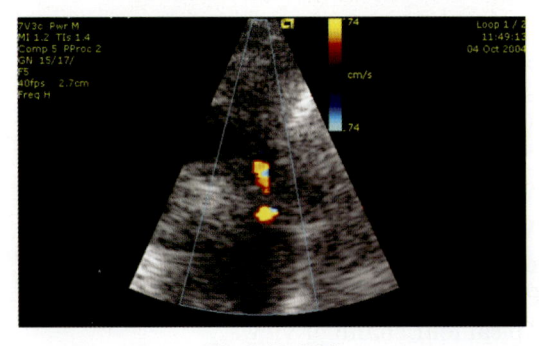

Fig. 5.12: PDA

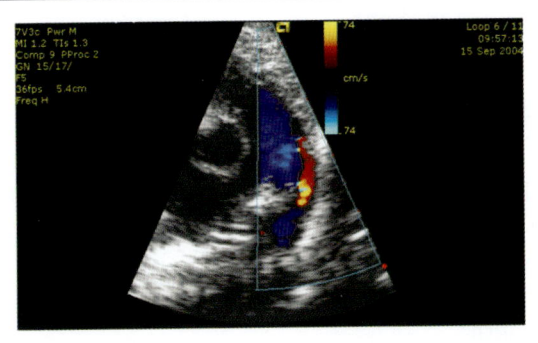

Fig. 5.13: Color flow in PDA

- The ductus may be short or long, straight or tortuous.
- Doppler performed on PA proximal to ductal opening. The peak velocity will give the pressure difference between aorta and PA (Fig. 5.14).

Clinical Manifestations

- In a small ductus patients are asymptomatic.
- Large ductus frequent respiratory infections, atelectasis and CHF may occur.

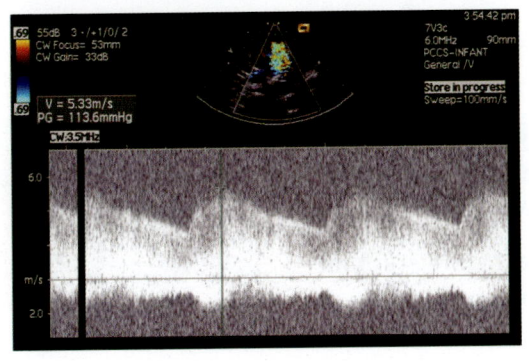

Fig. 5.14: PDA Doppler flow

ECG and X-ray chest findings are similar to those of VSD.

Echocardiography

- View
  - High transverse parasternal
  - Suprasternal.
- Diagnostic criteria
  - Lumen of the vessel visualized along the entire length
  - LAE
  - LV dilatation
  - Measure LA and LV reflecting the volume of left to right shunt
  - Look for associated defects like coarctation of aorta and aortopulmonary window.

Natural History

- Unlike PDA of prematures spontaneous closure of PDA does not occur. PDA of term are due to structural abnormality of ductal smooth muscle.
- PVOD, CHF or recurrent pneumonia.
- SBE, more frequent with small PDA.

PULMONARY STENOSIS (PS) (FIG. 5.15)

PS may be valvular, subvalvular (infundibular) or supravalvular.

Clinical Manifestations

- Mild PS children are asymptomatic.
- Moderate PS, dyspnea and easy fatiguability.
- Severe PS, heart failure, and exertional chest pain.

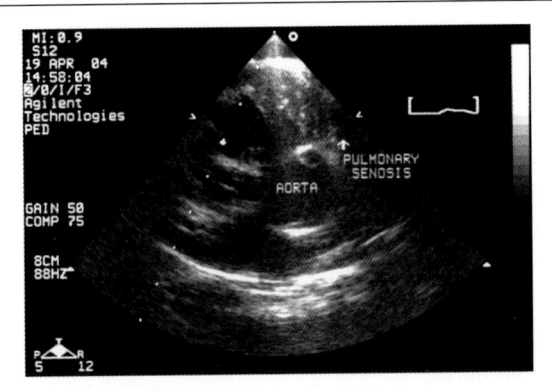

Fig. 5.15: Pulmonary stenosis

Echocardiography

- Views
  - Precordial short axis
  - High parasternal
  - Subxiphoid L4, S4.
- Diagnostic criteria
  - Doming of pulmonary valve during systole
  - Dilatation of main pulmonary artery
  - High velocity through MPA
  - In severe PS, R to L shunting may occur at PFO or ASD level.

Natural History

- Mild PS severity of stenosis is not progressive
- Moderate to severe PS it is progressive
- CHF may develop in severe stenosis
- SBE occasionally occurs
- Sudden death in severe stenosis.

CONGENITAL LEFT VENTRICULAR OUTFLOW OBSTRUCTION (LVOT)

Types

- Subvalvular
  - Discrete membranous stenosis
  - Fibromuscular tunnel.
- Valvular (Fig. 5.16)
  - Unicuspid
  - Bicuspid
  - Dysplastic.
- Supravalvular
  - Discrete (membranous or hourglass)
  - Aortic hypoplasia or atresia
  - Interrupted aortic arch
  - COA.

Subvalvular Stenosis

Echocardiography

- Views

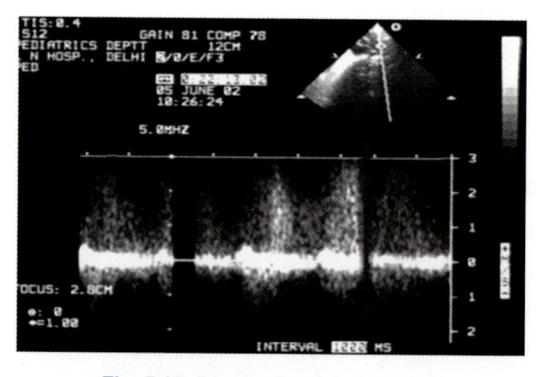

Fig. 5.16: Doppler flow in valvular AS

- Precordial long and short axis sweeps
- Apical two chamber view
- Subxyphoid L3, S3-5.
- Diagnostic criteria
  - Systolic flutter of aortic cusps (M-mode).
  - Membrane within the LVOT.
  - Anterior mitral leaflet fixed by a subaortic membrane.
  - Left ventricular hypertrophy.

AORTIC STENOSIS

Echocardiography

- Views
  - Precordial long and short axis
  - Right sternal border long and short axis
  - Subxiphoid L3.
- Diagnostic criteria
  - Systolic doming of aortic cusps during systole
  - LVH, aortic root dilatation
  - Diastolic flutter of AML
  - High velocity flow in ascending aorta.

Supravalvular Aortic Stenosis

- Views (older children)
  - Precordial long axis
  - Right sternal border long axis.

Features

- The lumen of the aorta is narrowed above the coronary ostia.

- Descending and ascending aorta may be hypoplastic.
- Left ventricular hypertrophy may be present.

Natural History

- Mild AS asymptomatic.
- Severe AS heart failure in newborns, chest pain, syncope and sudden death.
- Pressure gradient increases with growth.
- Worsening of AR may occur in subaortic stenosis.
- SBE is 4% in valvar AS.

COARCTATION OF AORTA (FIG. 5.17)

- 8–10% of all CHD.
- 30% of Turner's syndrome
- 85% of COA have bicuspid valve.

Clinical Manifestations

- Poor feeding, dyspnea and poor weight gain, and acute circulatory shock in first 6 weeks.
- 20–30% of COA develop CHF by 3 months.

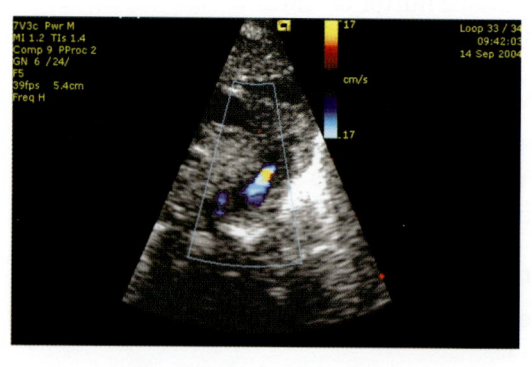

Fig. 5.17: Coarctation of aorta

Echocardiography

- Views
  - Subxiphoid L2
  - Suprasternal long axis.
- Diagnostic features
  - Aortic lumen is narrowed, typically distal to the left subclavian artery.
  - Hypoplastic aortic arch.
  - Poststenotic dilatation of the aorta.
  - Bicuspid aortic valve.
  - Doppler will show the severity of obstruction.
  - Bicuspid valve may cause stenosis or regurgitation with age.
  - SBE may occur on either aortic valve or on coarctation.
  - LV failure, rupture of aorta, hypertensive encephalopathy may develop during childhood.

chapter 6

Cyanotic Heart Disease

TRANSPOSITION OF GREAT ARTERIES (FIG. 6.1) (D-TGA)

- 5% of all CHDs
- M>F.

Pathology

In D-TGA aorta arises anteriorly from RV carrying desaturated blood to the body, and the PA arises posteriorly from LV carrying oxygenated blood to lungs. VSD is present in 30–40% of the patients with TGA.

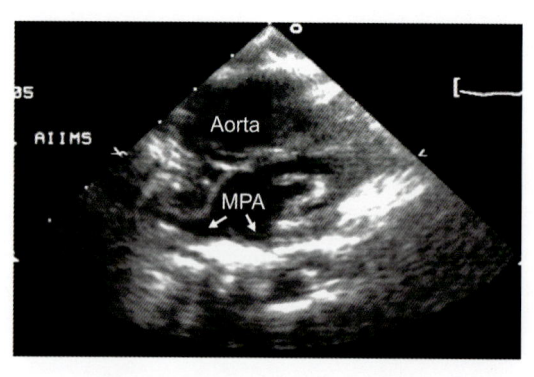

Fig. 6.1: TGA subxiphoid short axis

LVOT may be present in 30% patients of D-TGA with VSD.

Clinical Manifestations

- Cyanosis may be present from birth
- Signs of CHF with dyspnea and feeding difficulties during newborn period.

ECG

- RVH present after first few days of life.
- CVH may be present in infants with large VSD, PDA, or PVOD because all these conditions produce additional LVH.

X-ray chest

- Cardiomegaly with increased pulmonary vascularity.
- Superior mediastinal narrowing with egg-shaped cardiac silhouette.

Echocardiography

- Views
  - Subxiphoid S4–5, L3.
- Diagnostic findings
  - Pulmonary artery arising from the left ventricle-subxiphoid L3 demonstrates the right and left branching pattern of this vessel.
  - Aorta arising from right ventricle (subxiphoid S4).
  - Ventricles are identified by atrioventricular valves and papillary muscle morphology. Great arteries are identified by their branching pattern. ASD, VSD or PDA may be present.

– Parasternal short axis view shows great arteries in "double circles" instead of circle and sausage appearance.

Natural History

CHF occurs in first few weeks of life with progressive hypoxia and acidosis. Balloon atrial septostomy should be done when the septum is intact. Patients with VSD are the least cyanotic but most likely to develop CHF and PVOD. Patients with VSD and PS may have a long survival.

L-TGA

L-TGA occurs in 1% of all CHD.

Pathology

Visceroatrial relationship is normal, i.e. RA is to the right of LA. However, there is ventricular inversion, i.e. RV is located to the left of LV and LV is located to the right of RV. Great arteries are transposed with aorta arising from the RV and the PA rising from the LV. In 50% of the cases this is associated with dextrocardia. There are no functional abnormalities excepting VSD in 80%, PS (valvular) in 50% and tricuspid regurgitation in 30% of the cases.

Clinical Manifestation

Patients are asymptomatic when not associated with other lesions. Symptoms that develop are due to the associated defects.

ECG

Absence of Q waves in 1, V5, and V6 and or the presence of Q waves in V4R, or V1 is characteristic of the condition. Varying degree of AV block is common.

Atrial and/ventricular hypertrophy may be common.

X-ray chest

Straight, left upper cardiac border, formed by ascending aorta is a characteristic finding.

Associated cardiac lesions, may present its relevant cardiac findings.

Echocardiography

Features

- Parasternal long axis view is made by a more vertical and leftward scan, than with a normal heart.
- Parasternal short axis shows a double circle instead of normal circle and sausage pattern.
- In apical and subcostal four chamber views, LA is connected to tricuspid valve with a more apical attachment to the ventricular septum and the RA is connected to the mitral valve.

Clinical course is determined by presence or absence of associated defects and its complications.

TETRALOGY OF FALLOT (FIGS 6.2A AND B)

TOF occurs in 10% of all CHDs. It is the commonest cyanotic heart defect seen beyond infancy.

Pathology

It comprises of large VSD, RV outflow tract obstructions, RVH, and overriding of aorta.

The VSD in TOF is perimembranous with extension into pulmonary region.

RVOT is in form of infundibular stenosis (45%). In most serious anomaly the pulmonary valve is atretic (15%). The obstruction is rarely at pulmonary valve level.

Associated anomalies TOF occur in 25% of cases.

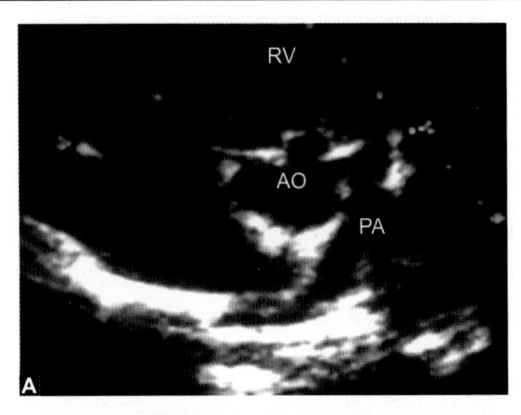

Fig. 6.2A: CP short axis

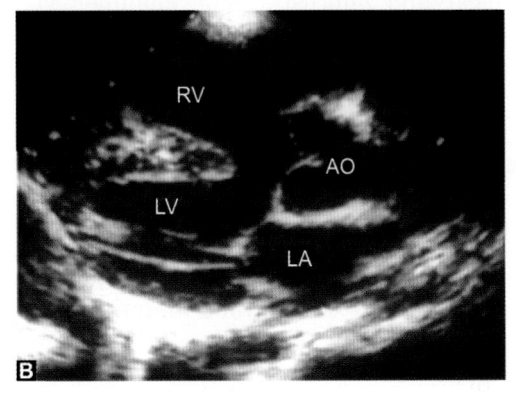

Fig. 6.2B: P long axis

Clinical Manifestations

- A heart murmur is audible at birth.
- Many patients are symptomatic with cyanosis at birth. Dyspnea on exertion, squatting, hypoxic spells develop later in mildly cyanotic infants.
- Patients with acyanotic TOF may be asymptomatic or may show signs of CHF from large left to right.

- Shunts.
- Cyanosis at birth may be present in TOF with pulmonary valve atresia.

ECG

RAD (+120° to +150°) is present in cyanotic TOF. In acyanotic, TOF QRS is normal.

RVH is usually present CVH is seen in acyanotic form.

X-ray chest

Cyanotic TOF

- Heart size is normal or smaller than normal, PVM's are reduced.
- Concave MPA segment with a boot-shaped heart.

Acyanotic TOF

- X-ray findings of acyanotic TOF are similar to small to moderate sized VSD.

Echocardiography

Views

Narrowed RVOT subxiphoid L4 and S4 (Fig. 6.2A)
Doppler shows the pressure gradient across the pulmonary valve

- Overriding aorta with large perimembranous VSD subxiphoid S3.
- Precordial long axis (Fig. 6.2B).

Natural History

Hypoxic spells occur depending on the severity of RVOT, and thereby growth retardation may develop in future.

Infants who are acyanotic at birth may become cyanosed later in infancy.

Brain abscess, cerebrovascular accidents and SBE are common complications.

Since central cyanosis predisposes to polycythemia—Iron deficiency anemia and coagulopathy should be remembered as potent complications.

TRICUSPID ATRESIA (FIGS 6.3A AND B)

Tricuspid atresia accounts for 1–3% of all CHDs.

Pathology

The tricuspid valve is absent, and RV is hypoplastic with absence of inflow portion of the RV. The associated defects such as ASD, VSD or PDA are necessary for survival.

Tricuspid atresia is usually classified according to the presence or absence of PS and TGA. The great arteries are normally related in 70% of cases and transposed in 30%. Transposition usually appears in complete form. In 3% of cases congenitally corrected form of transposition occurs. Coarctation of aorta is a frequently associated anomaly.

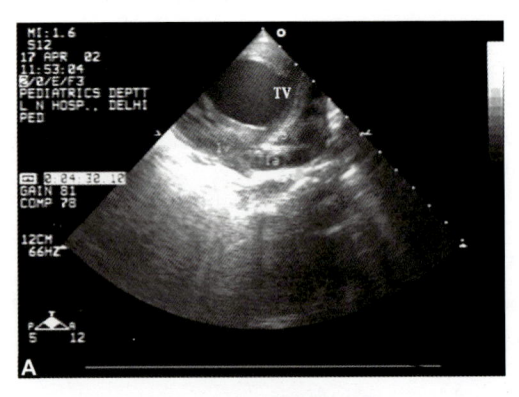

Fig. 6.3A: Subxiphoid (long axis)

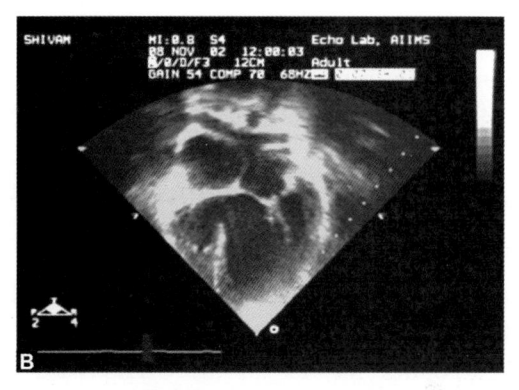

Fig. 6.3B: Apical (short axis)

Clinical Manifestations

- Cyanosis in severe form with occasional hypoxic spells.
- Tachypnea and poor feeding during infancy.

ECG

- Superior ORS axis (between 0–90°)
- LVH is usually present with RAH or sometimes combined atrial hypertrophy.

Echocardiography

- Absence of tricuspid orifice, there is a band present instead of TV(Fig. 6.6) valve marked hypoplasia of RV and a large LV in subxiphoid L2, S2.
- Apical four chamber view.
- Bulging of atrial septum towards left and size of ASD.
- Size of VSD, presence and severity of PS and presence of TGA should be looked for.

Natural History

Few infants with tricuspid atresia with normally related great arteries survive beyond 6 months without surgical palliation.

Some develop CHF because of increased blood flow.

Those who survive for the first 10 years, chronic volume overload of LV leads on to secondary cardiomyopathy.

TOTAL ANOMALOUS PULMONARY VENOUS RETURN (TAPVR) (FIG. 6.4)

TAPVR accounts for 1% of all CHDs with a male preponderance (4:1).

Pathology

The pulmonary veins instead of draining into LA, drain anomalously into either the systemic veins or into the

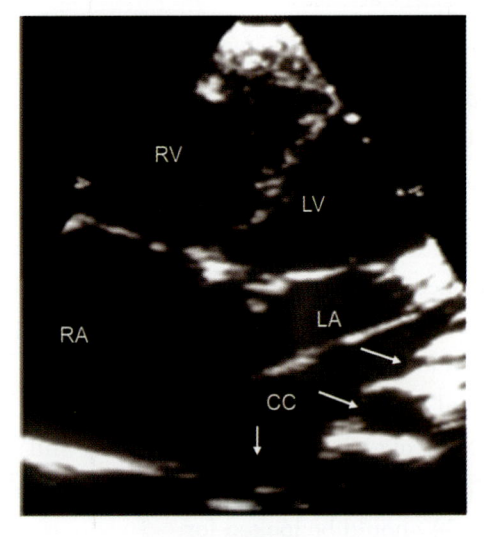

Fig. 6.4: TAPVR

RA. Depending on the drainage site, the defect may be divided into 4 types.

a. Supracardiac – 50% of TAPVR patients. The common pulmonary venous sinus drain into SVC and left innominate vein.
b. Cardiac 20% of TAPVR. Drainage takes place into the RA or coronary sinus.
c. Infracardiac–(subdiaphragmatic): 20% of TAPVR. Drainage is into portal vein, ductus venosus, hepatic vein or IVC. The common pulmonary vein penetrates the diaphragm to drain.
d. Mixed type 10% is a combination of all other types.

An interatrial communication (ASD or PFO) is necessary for survival.

The left side of the heart is relatively small.

Clinical Manifestations

- In TAPVR without pulmonary venous obstruction history of frequent chest infections with CHF leading on to growth retardation in infancy.
- History of mild cyanosis may be present in TAPVR with pulmonary venous obstruction. There is marked cyanosis and respiratory distress in the neonatal period leading to severe growth failure.

ECG

RVH of the volume overload type (rSR') with occasional RAH.

X-ray studies

Moderate to marked cardiomegaly with increase PVMs. "*Snowman*" sign or figure 8 configurations may be seen in supracardiac type.

Echocardiography

Views

- Atrial Anatomy—Subxiphoid L2
- Venous return— 1 subxiphoid L3 with coronal angulation.

Diagnostic criteria

- Entrance of pulmonary veins to right heart is demonstrated.
- Absence of pulmonary venous return to small LA.
- R to L shunt at PFO or ASD.
- Right ventricular dilatation.

TRUNCUS ARTERIOSUS (FIG. 6.5)

Truncus arteriosus is rare (occurs in less than 1% CHDs).

Pathology

Only a single trunk with a truncal valve—gives rise to systemic, pulmonary and coronary circulations (Fig. 6.6A). A large perimembranous VSD is usually present and truncal valve may be bicuspid, tricuspid or quadricuspid (Fig. 6.6B) and is often regurgitant.

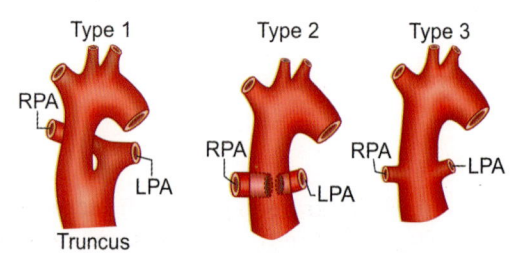

Fig. 6.5: Truncus arteriosus

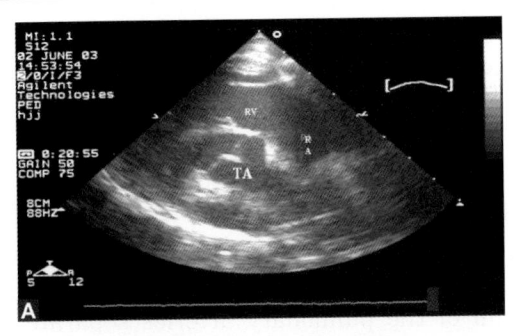

Fig. 6.6A: Parasternal long axis

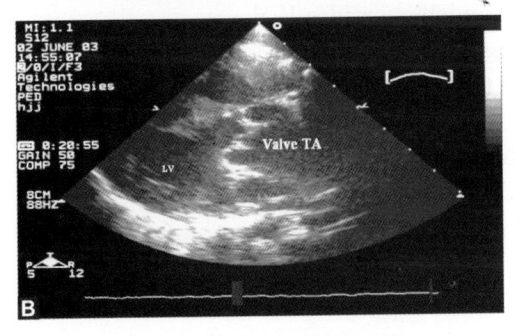

Fig. 6.6B: Parasternal long axis

Associated coronary artery abnormalities are common. Right-sided aortic arch is seen in 40% of patients.

Clinical Manifestations

- Cyanosis is present at birth.
- Signs of CHF also appear in the first few weeks after birth, with respiratory distress. These infants die of CHF by 6–12 months.
- If PVOD supervene by 6 months, child survives till 3rd decade. Commonly presents as a undernourished child in CHF, cyanosed with bounding peripheral pulses.

- A loud harsh murmur at lower parasternal border suggestive of VSD.

Echocardiography

Views

- Subxiphoid L3–4, S3–4.

Diagnostic criteria

- Origin of the pulmonary arteries separate or by a trunk from the ascending portion of single arterial root which overrides IVS.
- A high subtruncal VSD.
- The truncal valve is often redundant or thickened.
- The LA and LV are dilated.
- Other findings
  - LA and LV usually dilated
  - Truncal valve often redundant.

chapter 7

Acquired Valvular Disease

Echocardiography has become the examination of choice for evaluating valvular heart disease. 2-D echo provides an excellent tomographic examination of all the cardiac valves. M-mode records the subtle motion of the individual valves. Doppler evaluates the hemodynamic status of the valves. Stenotic and regurgitant valves are detected by abnormal flow pattern and color imaging.

RHEUMATIC HEART DISEASE

Given that echocardiography now provides the opportunity for enhancing early detection of subclinical RHD and thus potentially prevention of advanced disease, the establishment of optimal criteria for echocardiography-based diagnosis is essential.

RHD remains the main origin of heart valve disease in developing world. In these areas, it is recommended that significant subclinical valve lesions be labeled as probable RHD until proven otherwise and that affected children have long-term follow-up studies and be placed on secondary rheumatic fever prophylaxis. In 2001, a World Health Organization (WHO) Expert Committee established a consensus for the echocardiographic diagnosis of subclinical RHD based on the detection of valvular regurgitation by Doppler interrogation of the cardiac valves. Specific criteria for grading the severity of such regurgitation were included to allow the distinction between pathological versus physiological regurgitation and thus the diagnosis of subclinical RHD. However, the boundary between physiological valve regurgitation and authentic but minimal rheumatic lesions remains difficult to discern in some cases. Pathophysiologically, repeated rheumatic carditis can result in subvalvular or valvular thickening before the development of leaflet retraction and thereby regurgitation. Thus, we have previously proposed that morphological changes of valves affected by the rheumatic inflammatory process, even before the development of pathological regurgitation, likely indicate subclinical RHD, which might benefit from identification and thence secondary prevention.

Mitral Valve (MV) Anatomy and Function

The MV is located between left atrium (LA) and left ventricle (LV). The MV is a thin flexible structure and has 3 main components:
- 2 leaflets anterior and posterior.
- Chordae tendineae attached to papillar muscle (subvalvular apparatus).
- Annulus (valve ring).

The two leaflets are attached at one end to the annulus and at the other (free) edge at the chordae which are fixed to the LV wall by papillary muscle. The chordae holds each of the MV leaflets like cords hold a parachute canopy. The leaflets free edges meet at 2 points called the commissure. The area of mitral leaflets is about 2.5 times the area of the orifice at the annular level.

MITRAL STENOSIS (MS) (FIG. 7.1)

This is classified into congenital and acquired. Congenital MS is very rare. It may be associated with connective tissue disorders and collagen tissue disorders. Almost all acquired valvular diseases are rheumatic in origin.

Pathology

Rheumatic fever if autoimmune in origin caused by antibodies to streptococcal bacterial antigen found in heart. In acute stage there is inflammation of all the layers of the heart (pancarditis) thickening of the leaflets and fusion of the commissures. The left atrium and right side of heart chambers become dilated and hypertrophied. Severe pulmonary venous hypertension, congestion, and edema bring about alveolar wall fibrosis, loss of lung compliance and hypertrophy of pulmonary arterioles.

Clinical Manifestations

- Normal mitral valve is 4–6 cm^2. Symptoms begin to develop when the valve stenosis comes down to an

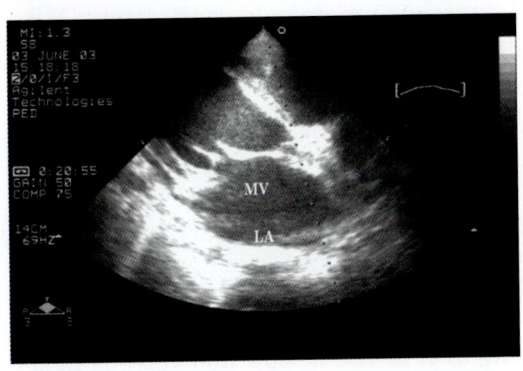

Fig. 7.1: Mitral stenosis parasternal long axis

area of 1.5 cm^2 and usually become severe once the area is less than 1 cm^2.
- The common manifestations in moderate to severe cases include fatigue, palpitations and exertional dyspnea with cough and hemoptysis occasionally.
- When the disease advances presence of RV dominance with weak peripheral pulses and elevated jugular venous pressure gradually supervene.
- Classical auscultatory findings are:
  - Loud opening snap in early diastole when the diseased valve snaps open forcibly by the high pressure in LA.
  - Similarly loud S2 when AV valves close forcibly.
  - Opening snap is followed by a mid-diastolic murmur.
  - Pansystolic murmur of tricuspid regurgitation is present in moderate to severe cases of MS.

Diagnosis

X-ray studies

- Left atrial dilatation and right ventricular hypertrophy with prominent main pulmonary artery (MPA).
- Lung fields show pulmonary venous congestion.
- Interstitial edema (Kerly B lines).
- Redistribution of PBF to the upperlobes.

ECG

RAD, LAH, RVH (due to pulmonary artery hypertension) Atrial fibrillation common in chronic MV disease.

Echocardiography

- Filling of ventricle is slow and valve is held open by persistent pressure gradient between LA and LV.

Acquired Valvular Disease 83

- Early diastolic or E to F closure is slower thus the mid-diastolic closing velocity of the valve or E to F slope is diminished.
- 2-D echo
  - Evaluates valvular morphology in MS.
  - Doming of AML in diastole. Doming indicates that the valve cannot accommodate all blood available for delivery in diastole.
  - MV assumes shape of a funnel.
  - Dilated LA along with dilated MPA, RV, and RA.

Natural History

Most children with mild to moderate MS are asymptomatic but become symptomatic on exertion. Atrial flutter or fibrillation accompanies chronic MS. SBE can occur as a rare complication.

MITRAL REGURGITATION (FIG. 7.2)

Mitral regurgitation (MR) is the most common valvular involvement in children with rheumatic heart disease.

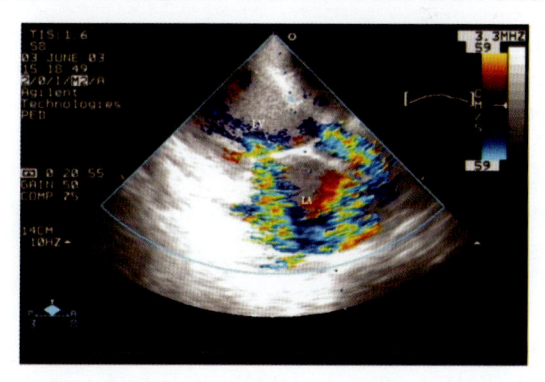

Fig. 7.2: Mitral regurgitation parasternal long axis

Pathology

Mitral valve leaflets are shortened because of fibrosis. When the degree of MR increases, LA and mitral valve ring gets dilated, which leads on to leakage of blood through MV into LA during ventricular systole. It ranges between very mild to very severe, when the majority of the LV volume empties into the LA than into the aorta, with each cardiac cycle.

Clinical Manifestations

- Mild to moderate cases in childhood are mostly asymptomatic. Rarely fatigue and palpitation are the manifestations.
- In severe MR, hyperdynamic pulsatile precordium—Exertional dyspnea, palpitation indicate CHF.
- A soft or absent first heart sound, loud second sound and third sound are heard.
- A regurgitant systolic murmur radiating to back are heard.

ECG

- Mild cases ECG is normal.
- Severe cases LVH with LAH, with occasional atrial fibrillation.

X-ray chest

- LA and LV enlargement depending on severity.

Echocardiography

- 2-D echo:
  - Mitral valve morphology
  - Flail MV leaflets and AML prolapse/vegetation

- Dilated LV with rapid filling.
- Septal and posterior wall motion becomes more vigorous.
- Color flow and Doppler: LA size increased mitral regurgitation jet is seen.

Pulmonary venous congestion may develop if pulmonary edema or CHF supervene.

Chronic MR

- Volume overload of LV dilatation with hyperdynamic movement.
- Volume overload of LA with dilatation.
- Large regurgitation refers to volume of it <4m/sec.
- Abnormal valve function, vegetation, prolapse, etc.

Natural History

- Patients are relatively stable for a long time but MS eventually supervenes.
- Pulmonary hypertension and LV failure may occur.
- Infective endocarditis is a rare complication.

MITRAL VALVE PROLAPSE

Mitral valve prolapse (MVP) is the most common valvular heart disease in industrialized nations affecting approximately 3–5% of population—At large, mostly in older children and adolescents and M:F=1:2.

MVP is an autosomal dominant genetically transmitted disease.

Etiology

Mitral valve prolapse (MVP) is idiopathic in more than 50% of cases.

- CHD is present in 1/3rd patients with MVP.
- ASD is a common defect, VSD and Ebstein's anomaly is associated rarely.
- Of all patients with MVP, 4% have Marfan's syndrome and nearly all patients with Marfan's have MVP.

MVP is familial in the primary form with an autosomal dominant mode of inheritance.

Clinical Manifestations

- MVP is usually asymptomatic but history of nonexertional chest pain or palpitation may be present.
- Occasional family history of MVP is present.
- Asthenic built with a high incidence of thoracic skeletal anomalies (80%), including pectus excavatum (50.8%), straight back syndrome (20%) and scoliosis.
- Typical auscultatory findings are midsystolic click with or without late systolic murmur best heard at apex. The click and murmur may be made more prominent by held expiration, left decubitus or leaning forward position.

ECG

Inverted T-waves in lead II, III and AVF occurs in 20–60% of patients.
- Arrhythmias.
- SVT and conduction disturbances are rarely reported.
- LVH or LAH is rarely present.

X-ray studies

- X-ray films are unremarkable except for LA enlargement in severe MR.

Echocardiography

- M-mode echo mid to lateral posterior excertion (>3 mm) of posterior and or anterior leaflet is considered diagnostic.
- 2-D echo more reliable. Parasternal long axis view shows prolapse of one or both.
- Mitral valve leaflets into the left atrium.
- MV leaflets may be thick and MR is occasionally demonstrated by color flow mapping and Doppler examination (Fig. 7.3).
- MVP is a progressive disease with less than full manifestation in children.

Natural History

MVP in children is asymptomatic with no restriction of activity.

Complications in adults like sudden death, and stroke, progressive MR, rupture of chordae tendineae, arrhythmias, and conduction disturbances may occur.

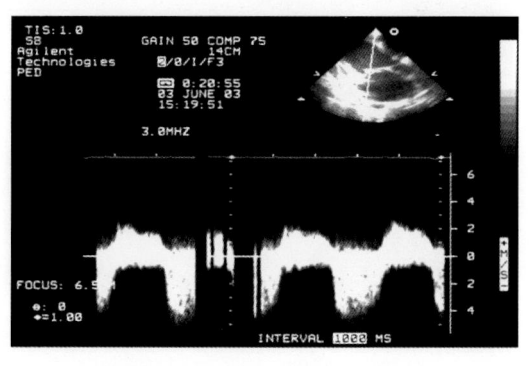

Fig. 7.3: Mitral regurgitation Doppler

Flail Mitral Valve

A flail mitral valve is best detected in 2-D echocardiography. The flail leaflet is a thickened valve in diastole. In systole, the diseased leaflet protrudes into left atrium, with tip of leaflet pointing towards left atrium. The most common cause of flail leaflet is ruptured chordae tendineae followed by ruptured papillary muscle.

AORTIC REGURGITATION (FIG. 7.4)

Aortic valve involvement in rheumatic heart disease results in aortic regurgitation, because by the time aortic stenosis develops, the patient is well beyond the pediatric age group. Though pure AR is less common than MR, and has been documented in 5–8%, most patients with AR have associated mitral valve disease.

Pathology

Semilunar cusps are deformed and shortened, and the valve ring is dilated so that cusps fail to appose tightly. The commissure are fused to a certain degree.

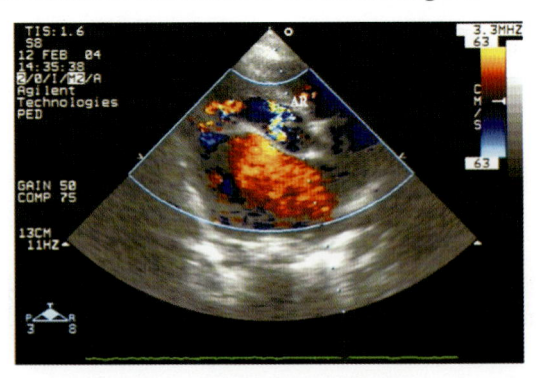

Fig. 7.4: Aortic regurgitation

Clinical Manifestations
- Patients with mild AR are usually asymptomatic.
- Moderate to severe AR palpitations with exercise intolerance with occasional chest pain leading to CHF.
- On examination there are features of hyperdynamic circulation—Pulsatile apex with intercostal pulsations and a wide pulse pressure.
- On auscultation: High pitched decrescendo murmur, heard best in 3rd and 4th left intercostals space. A mid-diastolic rumble at mitral area when AR is severe.
- Peripheral manifestations of wide pulse pressure in severe AR.
    - Prominent carotid pulsations
    - Pistol shot over femorals
    - Wide pulse pressure over radial arteries.

Natural History
- Patients remain asymptomatic for a long time.
- Anginal pain with CHF and associated arrhythmias are unfavorable signs.
- Infective endocarditis is a rare complication.

ECG
- In mild cases—Normal.
- In severe and prolonged—AR, LVH and LAH are both present.

X-ray chest
- Cardiomegaly because of LV dilatation in severe AR.
- Pulmonary venous congestion when LV dysfunction sets in.

Echocardiography

- LV diastolic dimension is proportional to the severity of AR.
- Color flow and Doppler gives an estimate of severity of AR.
  - Transducer is at apex.
  - Sample volume is in LVOT.
  - High velocity color flow.
  - *2-D echo*—Reverse doming of mitral leaflet.
  - *Doppler* is above the baseline and towards the transducer (Fig. 7.5).
  - *Pulsed Doppler* used to quantitate flow by measuring aortic flow and mitral flow and subtracting the two.

TRICUSPID REGURGITATION (FIGS 7.6A TO C)

Seen in 20% patients of rheumatic heart disease. It is difficult to differentiate between organic and functional regurgitation.

Clinical Manifestations

- There are no specific symptoms.

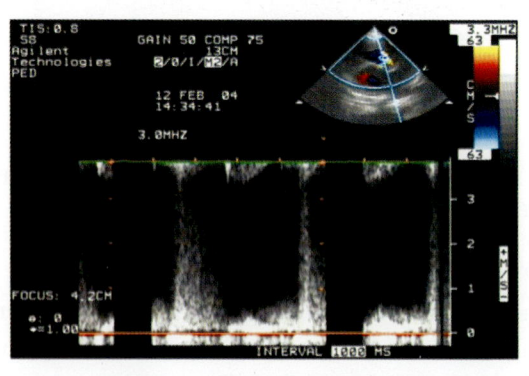

Fig. 7.5: Aortic regurgitation Doppler

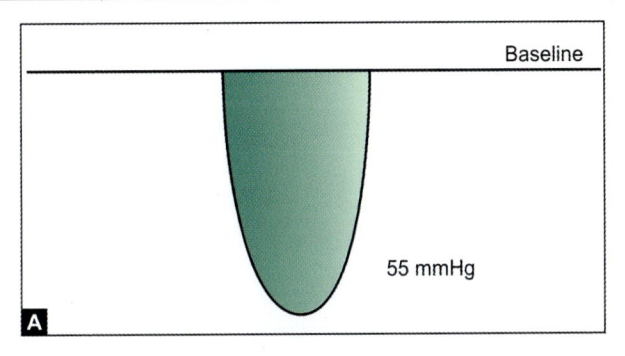

Fig. 7.6A: Tricuspid regurgitation

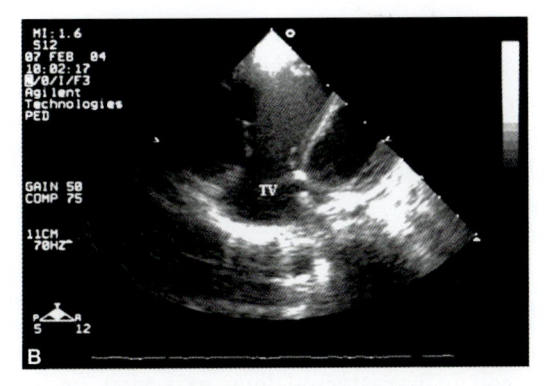

Fig. 7.6B: Tricuspid regurgitation

- Pain in right hypochondrium due to congested liver.
- Fatigue due to decreased systolic output.
- Systolic pulsation on liver.
- Systolic murmur in the lower right sternal border increasing in intensity during inspiration.

ECG

- Shows right ventricular hypertrophy.

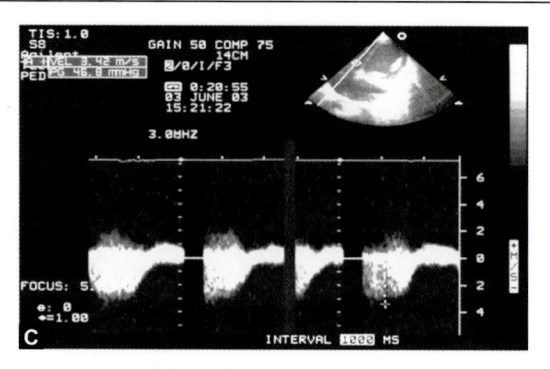

Fig. 7.6C: Tricuspid regurgitation Doppler

- Echocardiography and Doppler can document and quantitate severity of TR.
- Severity of tricuspid regurgitation depends on size of TR jet and color flow image.
- 2-D shows dilated RV and flattening of IVS during diastole.
- M-mode shows dilated RV.

TRICUSPID STENOSIS

The hallmark of this disease is doming of the tricuspid valve, seen in parasternal long axis view or in apical four-chamber view. In addition to doming, thickening of leaflets and restricted motion helps in diagnosis of tricuspid stenosis. The M-mode and Doppler recording are similar to that of mitral stenosis.

chapter 8

Cardiac Infections

INFECTIVE ENDOCARDITIS

Infective endocarditis (IE) is one of the most dreaded complications of structural heart disease. Over the years the advent of echocardiography and further development and refinement of echocardiographic techniques have contributed to a better diagnosis and management of endocarditis. More precise criteria for the diagnosis of IE have been established that assist physicians in making a more objective assessment of the varied clinical manifestations of this process.

Definition

Infective endocarditis is a microbial infection of the endocardial surface of the heart (Fig. 8.1). Native or prosthetic valves are the most frequently involved sites but can also involve septal defects, mural endocardium or intravascular foreign devices such as intracardiac patches, surgically corrected shunts and intravenous catheter. Endocarditis remains an important complicating factor in patients with rheumatic valvular disease. 70% of the IE is a complication of congenital heart disease. Neonatal IE has been reported in large number of cases with structurally normal heart on right side. Use of prosthetic intravascular catheter is a common association.

The risk of endocarditis in general population is 5 cases per 100,000 persons. In high-risk group the incidence is substantially higher (300–2160 cases per 100,000 persons).

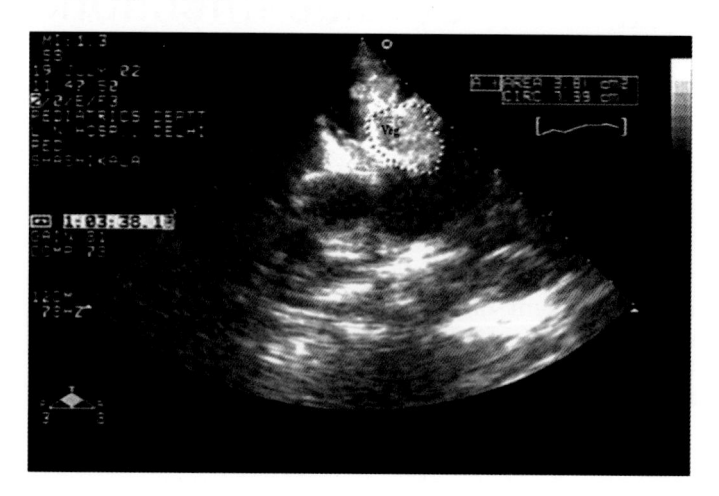

Fig. 8.1: Vegetation on tricuspid valves

Pathology

The greater the turbulence of flow, around the cardiac lesion, e.g. VSD, higher is the risk of infective endocarditis. This is because of endothelial damage results in platelet and fibrin deposition, which can subsequently become infected to form vegetations. A vegetation is usually found in the low-pressure side of the defect either around the defect or on the opposite surface of jet. Effect of the flow damages the endothelium. Vegetations are found in the pulmonary artery in patent ductus arteriosus or systemic PA shunts or on the atrial surface of mitral valve in mitral regurgitation and ventricular surface of aortic valve.

Review of literature over the past three decades the most common organisms are *α-hemolytic (viridans) streptococci* followed by *staphylococci*. Gram-negative bacteria cause less than (10%) of endocarditis in children.

Clinical Manifestation

History

- History of underlying cardiac defect in 10%.
- History of toothache or dental procedure.
- Fever (90%) low grade or high with headache, malaise, lack of appetite.
- History of complications hematuria, convulsions.
- Physical examination.
- Presence of heart murmur, depending on the defect.
- Splenomegaly 70%.
- Manifestation of heart failure.
- Skin manifestations—Petechiae in 50%.
- Embolic phenomena.
- Pulmonary emboli in patients with VSD, PDA, etc.
- Hemiparesis, renal failure, Roth spots/retinal hemorrhages.

Laboratory investigations

- Positive blood culture in 90%. Three samples for cultures are taken from different venipuncture sites after aseptic precautions because bacteremia is continuous and antimicrobials have to be started at the earliest.
- Acute phase reactants—Elevated.

- Anemia with leukocytosis with a shift to the left.
- Erythrocyte sedimentation rate elevated.
- Hematuria microscopic in 30%.

Echocardiography

- Two-dimensional echocardiographic examinations demonstrate vegetations more than 3 mm in diameter.
- The echocardiographic diagnosis of vegetation is finding of echogenic mass on valve leaflets. The M-mode shows shaggy echoes on valve leaflets. The vegetations on aortic valve leaflets are similar to those on mitral valve. The echoes from the vegetation may be seen best in either systole or in diastole, depending on direction of ultrasonic beam. An important complication of vegetation is the presence of abscess. The abscess frequently but not always has an echo-free center. It is important to know the extent of valve involved with the vegetation and the surrounding tissue.
- Vegetations may be detected on the different valves and in cyanotics the vegetations are mostly right-sided.
- When vegetations are not detected, it does not rule out IE and serial echo studies are indicated.
- When IE is suspected and echo evidence of vegetations may persist for months after complete cure.

PERICARDIAL DISEASE

The pericardium is a sac-like structure which surrounds the heart and consists of two layers with a potential space in between. The visceral layer—The inner serous layer is attached to the inner surface of the myocardium. The parietal layer—Outer fibrous layer, consists of elastic and collagen fibers. The pericardial space—It is a potential space separating the visceral and parietal layers and is lubricated with lymph which is less than 50 ml. Blood vessels, lymphatics and nerve fibers are beneath the visceral pericardium and surround the parietal pericardium.

Clinical Features

- Chest pain—Sharp associated with breathing.
- Friction rub—It is a grating, scratching sound caused by abrading of inflamed pericardial surface with cardiac motion. It is best heard in 2–4th intercostal spaces along left sternal border or along midclavicular line. It is loudest in upright position with patient leaning forward. Muffled heart sounds in the presence of large effusions.
- Ewart's sign—Subscapular dullness on percussion, due to compression of lung by massively enlarged heart. There may be abnormal breath sounds in that region.
- Cardiac tamponade—Features include low cardiac output, elevated central venous pressures, paradoxical pulses, muffled or diminished heart sounds and tachycardia.

X-ray chest

In acute pericarditis, heart size may be normal. In pericardial effusion, cardiac silhouette is considerably enlarged. Water bottle heart or triangular heart with smooth cut borders is seen in pericardial effusion.

Echocardiography

- Normal pericardial sac is a potential space and heart is in direct contact with surrounding structures.

- Presence of fluid enhances the diagnosis of pericardial effusion. However, its absence does not exclude pericarditis.

Thickened pericardium

- Pericardium is echogenic and adherent to the posterior ventricular wall.

Constrictive pericardium

- M-mode sign of constriction is the flattening of mid and late diastolic position of left ventricular free wall.
- Interventricular septal motion may be abnormal in patients with constrictive pericarditis.
- The principle finding is exaggerated anterior motion of septum with atrial filling. Because posterior wall of left ventricle cannot move freely, increase in left ventricle volume with atrial systole produces displacement of septum towards low pressure of right ventricle.
- 2-D echo shows a dilated inferior vena cava without respiratory variation.
- In presence of pericardial effusion, the pericardial space fills with relatively echo-free fluid, which separates heart from surrounding structure. In long axis as well as short axis fluid primarily collects posteriorly, anterior pericardial effusion is a smaller space and is not as free of near field clutters. Whether the heart floats or sinks depends on the amount of fluid.

Small effusion (Figs 8.2 and 8.3)

- Small echo: Free space posteriorly and hardly any fluid anteriorly.

- Moderate effusion: Large echo-free space posteriorly and small echo-free space anteriorly.
- Large effusion echo-free space that surrounds the heart.

2-D echo is essential for loculated effusion. Loculated pericardial fluid may be suspected when there is distention of oblique pericardial sinus behind left atrium. Sometimes, pleural effusion may be confused with pericardial effusion. In long axis view pericardial effusion tapers as it approaches the left atrium. Another differentiating point is that descending aorta is separated from the left atrium by pericardial effusion but not pleural effusion.

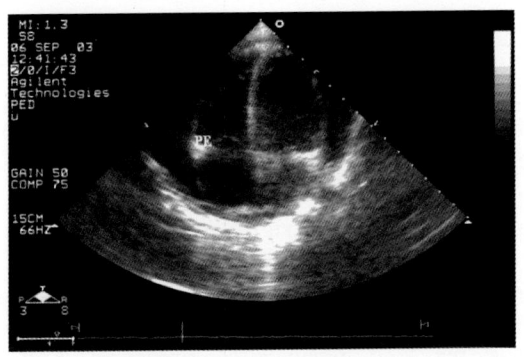

Fig. 8.2: Pericardial effusion

Quantification of pericardial fluid

- Effusions that totally surround the heart are at least 1 cm in width is designated as large effusion.
- A moderate effusion is one that surrounds the heart but is less than 1 cm at its greatest width.
- Small effusion is one that is localized posteriorly and is less than 1 cm in width.

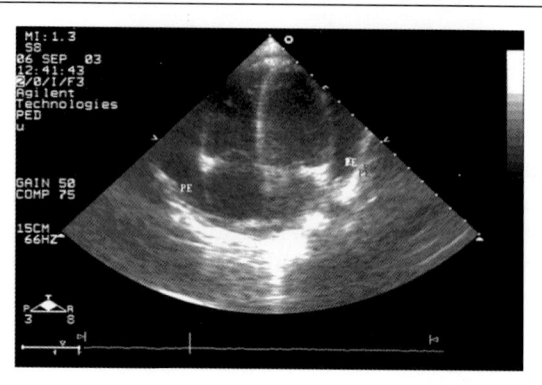

Fig. 8.3: Pleural effusion

Cardiac tamponade

- The most important sign is collapse of cardiac chambers in diastole. There is right ventricular and right atrial wall collapse in diastole. Timing of collapse can be made by correlating mitral valve opening or septal and posterior ventricular motion.
- Right ventricle and right atrial collapse is used for detecting cardiac tamponade. It is the right-sided chambers that collapse because these are low pressures chambers with thin walls collapsing under elevated pericardial pressure. Left atrial or left ventricular collapse is possible when fluid accumulates eccentrically or is loculated. Inferior vena cava plethora with blunted respiratory variation is an important sign of cardiac tamponade.
- "Swinging heart" requires a large chronically accumulated pericardial effusion with minimal adhesions.

chapter 9

Disease of Myocardium

CARDIOMYOPATHY

The term cardiomyopathy refers to any structural or functional abnormality of the ventricular myocardium not associated with coronary artery disease, high blood pressure, valvular, congenital heart disease or pulmonary vascular disease. They are broadly divided into two main categories primary and secondary. The latter is that where it is associated with a systemic disorder and is termed "specific heart muscle disease". Primary (idiopathic) Cardiomyopathies are classified into three main groups—Dilated (congestive), hypertrophic, and restrictive, which are further be classified based on underlying pathology.

Hypertrophic Cardiomyopathy (FIG. 9.1)

Hypertrophic cardiomyopathy (HCM) is a congenital disease that may manifest in infancy, childhood, adolescence or young adulthood. Recent studies have confirmed the genetic predisposition of HCM and with appropriate therapy; most patients can enjoy a reasonable lifestyle with little fear of sudden death.

Pathology

The most characteristic abnormality is hypertrophied

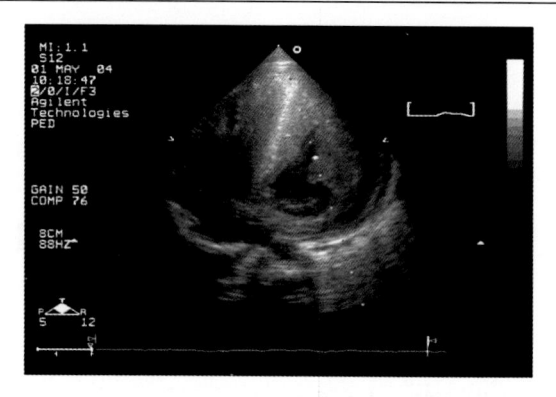

Fig. 9.1: Hypertrophic cardiomyopathy

LV, with ventricular cavity usually small or normal in size. Although asymmetric septal hypertrophy (ASM)— A condition formerly known as idiopathic hypertrophic subaortic stenosis is very common, the hypertrophy may be concentric or localized to a small segment of septum.

Microscopically an extensive disarray of hypertrophied myocardial cells and myocardial scarring may also occur. In some patients, an intracavitary pressure gradient develops during systole partly because of systolic anterior motion (SAM) of the mitral valve against the hypertrophied septum, which is called hypertrophic obstructive cardiomyopathy (HOCM). The SAM is probably created by the high outflow velocities and venturi forces. The myocardium itself has an enhanced contractile state, but diastolic ventricular filling is impaired by abnormal stiffness of the LV which may lead to LA enlargement and pulmonary venous congestion producing congestive symptoms (exertional dyspnea, orthopnea, paroxysmal nocturnal dyspnea). In 60% of cases, HCM appears to be genetically transmitted as an autosomal dominant trait and it occurs sporadically at rest.

Clinical manifestations

- The presentation of HCM in infancy can be very different from that of an older child. Easy fatiguability, dyspnea, palpitation and other signs of CHF may be presently manifesting as failure to thrive.
- Family history of HCM is positive in 30–60% of patients.
- Bradycardia and central cyanosis —Produced on crying.
- A sharp upstroke of arterial pulse is characteristic. A left ventricular heave and a systolic thrill at the apex may be present.
- An ejection systolic murmur of varying severity may be heard at the apex or along the left parasternal border.

Natural history

The obstruction due to hypertrophy may be absent, stable or slowly progressive. Genetically predisposed children often show an increasing wall thickness during childhood and adolescence. Progression of left ventricular hypertrophy may be seen in patients of second decade. Some adolescents manifest with symptoms of severe congestive heart failure, following a viral illness. Echocardiography reveals septal hypertrophy and left ventricular dilatation and markedly depressed left ventricular function.

ECG

- Left ventricular hypertrophy with strain pattern
- Abnormally deep Q-wave pattern (ST-T) wave changes
- Abnormal deep Q-waves/septal hypertrophy.

X-ray studies

- Mild left ventricular enlargement with a globular heart
- The pulmonary vascularity is normal.

Echocardiography

- Presence of right and left ventricular hypertrophy in infancy.
- A characteristic feature of HOCM is hypertrophy of IVS disproportionate to free wall of left ventricle. The four-chamber view is the best to identify hypertrophied IVS.
- Septal hypertrophy is characteristic of HOCM.
- 2-D echo demonstrates concentric hypertrophy, localized segmental hypertrophy or asymmetric septal hypertrophy.
- M-mode asymmetric septal hypertrophy of interventricular septum and occasionally systolic anterior motion (SAM) of anterior mitral leaflet in obstructive type.
- Patient with hypertension may produce hypertrophic cardiomyopathy or may exhibit asymmetric septal hypertrophy.
- Newborns of diabetic mother may mimic hypertrophic cardiomyopathy. Commonly hypertrophic cardiomyopathy may be accompanied by dynamic obstruction of LVOT.
- The echocardiographic hallmark is systolic anterior motion (SAM) of mitral valve.
- M-mode demonstrates motion of mitral valve apparatus towards IVS.
- Dynamic LVOT may have concentric hypertrophy.
- Pericardial effusion, anemia and hypovolemia may be associated with hypertrophic subaortic stenosis.

Mitral regurgitation may increase the early filling phase and is commonly present in hypertrophic cardiomyopathy.

Idiopathic Dilated Cardiomyopathy (Fig. 9.2)

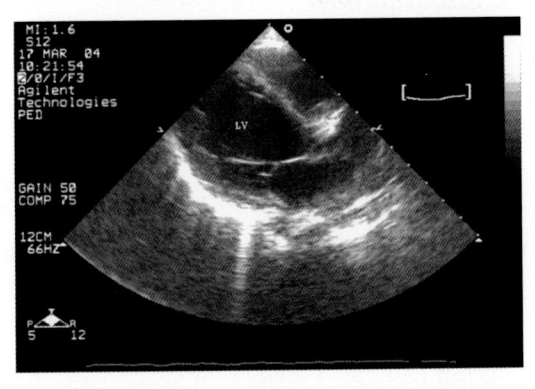

Idiopathic dilated cardiomyopathy (IDC) is a disease of infancy and more than 50% manifest before 2 years of age and the incidence is equal in both the genders. The etiology is unknown though familial incidence is equal in both genders. A hereditary basis has been documented.

Pathology

On postmortem examination there is enlargement and dilatation of all four-chambers, though the ventricles are more dilated than the atria. The development of left ventricular hypertrophy has a more protective role in dilated diastole, cardiomyopathy, presumably because it reduces the systolic wall stress and this protects against further cavity dilatation. Microscopically there is extensive areas of interstitial and perivascular fibrosis

Fig. 9.2: Idiopathic dilated cardiomyopathy

involving left ventricular subendocardium. No virus has been identified in tissues of DCM and no immunological, histochemical, morphological, ultrastructural, and biological dilatation. Microscopically there is extensive areas of interstitial and perivascular fibrosis involving left ventricular subendocardium. No virus has been identified in tissues of DCM and no immunological, histochemical, morphological, ultrastructural and biological markers have been diagnosis of idiopathic dilated cardiomyopathy.

Clinical picture

- Initial presentation is preceded by upper respiratory infection or gastroenteritis/gastritis in 35–50% of cases.
- Manifestation of congestive heart failure—Feeding difficulties, tachypnea, excessive perspiration leading to failure to thrive.
- Some present with ventricular or supraventricular tachycardia.

Physical examination

- Ill-looking child with moderate to severe respiratory distress.
- Moderate to severe pallor.
- Manifestation of low cardiac output state—Weak peripheral pulses with low blood pressure and narrowed pulse pressure.
- "Pulse alternans" a common finding where volume of each pulse alternates.
- Thoracic over distention and rarely prominence of left hemithorax.
- On auscultation—Muffled heart sounds with

presence of gallop rhythm. Initially murmurs are absent but soft apical pansystolic murmur of mitral regurgitation often appears after few days, once the cardiac function improves.
- Other signs of CHF—Enlarged tender liver, facial edema in an infant. Neck vein distention and pedal edema are rarely found in infants but frequently in older children and adolescents.

Laboratory investigations

Chest X-ray

Cardiomegaly secondary to dilatation of left atrium and left ventricle and presence of pulmonary venous congestion.

ECG

Sinus tachycardia with left ventricular hypertrophy and T-wave changes are seen in most of the patients.

Echocardiography

- Dilated and poorly contracting LV.
- LV is dilated and little difference between systole and diastole.
- Common finding is incomplete closure of MV and papillary muscle dysfunction.
- Pericardial effusion and intracavitary thrombus may be seen.
- Mitral inflow Doppler tracing demonstrates a reduced E velocity and decreased, E/A ratio compared to normal subjects.

Natural history

Progressive deterioration in clinical condition and about

60% die of intractable heart failure in 3–4 years after the onset of symptoms.

Atrial and ventricular arrhythmias develop during the course of the disease process.

Systemic or pulmonary embolism resulting from dislodgement of intracavitary thrombus.

Causes of death include congestive heart failure. Sudden death may also result from arrhythmias and massive embolization.

Restrictive Cardiomyopathy (Fig. 9.3)

Restrictive cardiomyopathy (RC) is an extremely rare cardiomyopathy in children.

Pathology

This condition is characterized by abnormal diastolic ventricular filling resulting from excessively stiff ventricular walls. The ventricles are neither dilated nor hypertrophied and contractility is normal. The atria are dilated and they resemble constrictive pericarditis in

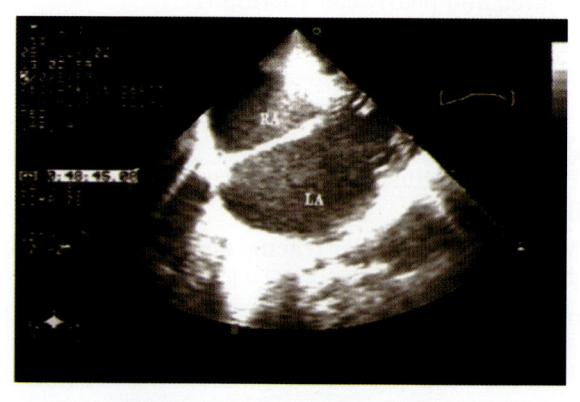

Fig. 9.3: Restrictive cardiomyopathy

clinical presentation and hemodynamic abnormalities. There may be areas of myocardial fibrosis or the myocardium may be infiltrated by various materials such as amyloidosis, sarcoidosis, hemochromatosis, glycogen deposits, etc.

Clinical manifestations

- History of exercise intolerance, weakness, exertional dyspnea or chest pain.
- Hepatomegaly, elevated jugular venous pressure, 'gallop rhythm', systolic murmur of TR or MR may be present.

Chest X-ray

Cardiomegaly and pulmonary congestion.

ECG

Shows paroxysms of SVT and atrial fibrillation.

Echocardiography

- Characteristic biatrial enlargement with normal sized LV.
- Contractility remains normal till late stages.
- Atrial thrombus may be present.
- Mitral inflow Doppler tracings shows an increased E velocity with decreased deceleration time and increased E/A ratio.
- Dilated LA and RA.
- Dilated poorly contracting left ventricle and echocardiographic signs of low cardiac output and high intracardiac pressures.
- The left ventricle is dilated with little difference in systole and diastole. All systolic indices, i.e. fractional

shortening, fractional area change and ejection fraction is reduced. Wall function remains normal and global dysfunction is generalized with increased left ventricular filling pressures and usually mitral regurgitation, LA dilatation is common.
- Mitral inflow is abnormal in patients with severe myocardial dysfunction. As mitral regurgitation or elevated left ventricular diastolic pressures occur, an abnormal relaxation pattern may progress towards abnormal compliance, with a tall E and small A-wave, which carries a poor prognosis.
- A common finding is incomplete closure of mitral valve or papillary muscle dysfunction. This contributes to MR. This occurs in number of disease states. Patients with an infiltrative cardiomyopathy such as amyloidosis, glycogen storage disease or thalassemia, produces this picture.
- The hallmark of restrictive physiology is abnormal compliance of left ventricle with rapid inflow and abrupt cessation of flow early in diastole. An early diastolic drop is followed by rise in left ventricular pressure giving the 'dip and plateau' or square root sign. The respiratory variation in flow velocities of tricuspid and mitral valves is minimal distinguishing it from constrictive pericarditis, which has a similar physiologic picture and greater respiratory variation. Doppler findings with restrictive cardiomyopathy can be subtle.
- With amyloidosis which is a classic example of restrictive cardiomyopathy, early stages of the disease, will produce abnormal left ventricular relaxation pattern with mitral flow pattern characterized by short E and tall A-wave, accompanied by hemodynamic factors such as mitral regurgitation, elevated filling pressures, elevated preload or afterload.

Infiltrative Cardiomyopathy

Cardiac muscle is infiltrated by abnormal substances, myocardial changes detected by echo include amyloidosis, iron overload from multiple transfusions, hemochromatosis, thalassemia, sarcoidosis, glycogen storage disease or Pompe's and mucolipidosis.

The most common infiltrative cardiomyopathy, in echodiagnosis is amyloid heart disease. Amyloid infiltrates the heart therefore there is thickening of myocardial walls and valves. There is hypertrophied interventricular septum and posterior left ventricular walls. Thickened interatrial septum is not common. Also there is minimal pericardial effusion. Left ventricle is not dilated; its systolic functions remain intact. Since filling of left ventricle is abnormal, thus left atrial dilatation occurs. The mitral flow of amyloid heart disease is restrictive type.

When there is reduced systolic function the prognosis is poor. Many of the infiltrative cardiomyopathies like a Pompe's produce nonspecific echo findings. The walls are thickened and echo reflective. Hypertrophic walls look like asymmetric or concentric hypertrophy. Neuromuscular dystrophies due to Friedreich's ataxia and Duchenne's may have echo findings of nonspecific hypertrophy like LVH or dysfunction, concentric hypertrophy, dilated cardiomyopathy, and asymmetric cardiomyopathy.

Infective agents

Viral infections, affecting the heart may cause dilated or hypertrophic cardiomyopathy. Regional wall motions can be affected also. Tuberculosis may cause restrictive cardiomyopathy. Patients with HIV, frequently have cardiac abnormalities, in form or dilated cardiomyopathy and pericardial effusion.

TRAUMA

This may affect the acoustic properties of the myocardium in form of disruption of a valve or wall, septal defects, pseudoaneurysm, ruptured papillary muscle in form of a valvular regurgitation.

Left ventricular thrombus may occur because of blunt chest trauma. Electric trauma may cause regional wall motion.

Systemic Illness

- Systemic hypertension may cause left ventricular hypertrophy with alteration of left ventricular systolic and diastolic function.
- Diabetics alter left ventricular diastolic function. Left ventricular hypertrophy, septal hypertrophy, and systolic anterior motion (SAM) may be identified in children of diabetic mother.
- Acromegaly produces cardiomegaly with concentric left ventricular hypertrophy.
- Hypothyroidism shows a reversible type of cardiomyopathy.
- Lupus erythematous produces pericardial effusion.
- Acute rheumatic fever produces myocarditis that involves not only valves but also myocarditis.

chapter 10
Pediatric Echocardiogram Report and its Pitfalls

Pitfall means something hidden or not immediately obvious.

Most of the echo report gives an accurate anatomic diagnosis. With the increasing expertise the need for catheterization and angiography is coming down. Proper interpretation needs help from history, clinical examination, chest X-ray, and ECG.

Echocardiography aims is to find out the physiological consequence of the anatomic defect and to formulate the therapy to correct it.

ERRORS

- Tworetzky, et al. (1999), reported a major diagnostic error of 2% in a group of 503 patients with complex CHD.
- Dorfman, et al. (2005), found a major error in 5.2% in LBW infants and 1.9% in others in a cohort of 570 children.
- Others reported a diagnostic error in 2–8% of cases.

Source of Pitfalls

Related to machine:
- Inadequate image quality

- Improper transducer or settings.

Inadequate assessment of relatively insignificant abnormality.
- Not following a segmental approach.
- And not assessing completely the possible associations.
- Pattern of reporting is not being followed.
- Technical proficiency is inadequate.

Common Difficulties

- Significance/severity of a lesion
- Associated anomaly
- Assessment of volume overload
- Ventricular function evaluation
- Assessment of valves and associated anomaly
- Evaluation of PAH
- Arch anomalies
- Flow across a shunt
- Great vessels anatomy
- Abnormal/extracardiac structures.

Significance of a Lesion, e.g. VSD

- VSD size may be erroneous to assess severity.
- To look for ventricular volume overload and extent of pulmonary hypertension.
- Gradient should be properly assessed and can be used for follow-up.
- Associated anomaly should be looked properly.

Small ASD with large right-sided volume overload— The lesions to be looked for are PAPVC, another ASD, Ebstein's, or significant PR.

Small VSD with high RV systolic pressure— need to look for RVOT.

LV volume overload / dysfunction

- Then look for L to R shunt not obviously visible
- Need to think of AP window
- Global/segmental hypokinesia
- Exclusion of coronary anomaly, aneurysm
- Have to look for coronary arising from PA.

Valves and associated anomaly

- Mitral valve anomalies are commonly missed.
- Need to look for LVOT, supravalvular aortic stenosis specially in presence of LVH.
- RVOT obstruction with valvular PS.
- Ebstein's anomaly in presence of low pressure TR.

Assessment of pulmonary artery hypertension (PAH)

- Unexplained PAH needs review again.
- Shunts may be missed because of PAH.
- Contrast study may be helpful.
- To look for cor-triatriatum, LA membrane, supramitral ring.
- Pulmonary vein stenosis may be the cause.

Arch anomalies

- Most commonly overlooked if clinical examination is not done.
- Peripheral pulses may be normal with interrupted aortic arch (IAA).
- Some anomalies are difficult to diagnose—like double aortic arch.

Flow across a shunt

- Proper assessment of flow by color Doppler and PW Doppler needed.

- Shunts flowing R to L may give clue to major anomaly like TAPVC.

How to avoid pitfalls?

- Segmental approach of echocardiography.
- Proper knowledge of associations.
- Giving stress in complete anatomic and physiologic diagnosis, crucial in the management.
- To evaluate history, clinical examination, chest X-ray, ECG, etc. before doing the echo.

chapter 11

Fetal Echocardiography

Fetal echocardiography is an ultrasonic evaluation of the fetal cardiovascular system. The optimal timing for performance of fetal echocardiogram is 18–22 weeks gestation. Beyond this the images are more difficult to form as the fetal body mass to amniotic fluid increases. A variety of maternal or fetal disorders may result in abnormality of the fetal cardiovascular system. In these circumstances a fetal echocardiogram should be performed. Congenital heart disease is the most common anomaly found in human.[1] As the detection rate of congenital anomaly increases, the demand for fetal echocardiography increases. It provides a smooth transition between the pre-and postnatal states, with the opportunity to provide immediate care at birth, thereby avoiding hemodynamic compromise. Fetal echocardiography can provide improved understanding when applied to cardiovascular abnormalities unrelated to congenital heart disease. Though it has been recommended to use four-chamber view as a part of obstetric examination, many a anomalies may go undiagnosed. Right and left ventricular outflow tract and great artery visualization allows a more effective screening of congenital heart disease.[2,3]

INDICATIONS

Maternal indications: Family history of CHD, metabolic disorders (diabetes, PKU), exposure to teratogens, exposure to prostaglandin inhibitors (ibuprofen, salicylic acid, indomethacin). Rubella infection, autoimmune disease like Sjögren's syndrome, systemic lupus erythematosus (SLE). Familial inherited disorders like Ellisvan Creveld, Marfan's, Noonan's syndrome and in vitro fertilization.

Fetal indications: Abnormal obstetric ultrasound screen, extracardiac abnormality, chromosomal abnormality, arrhythmias, hydrops, increased first trimester translucency. Multiple gestation and twin-twin transfusion syndrome.

EQUIPMENT

Ultrasound system performing fetal echocardiography should have capability for performing two-dimensional, M-mode, Doppler imaging. The requirement of fetal echocardiogram are more stringent than for an infant or child with congenital or acquired heart disease. Frame rates of 80–100 HTz are needed to view heart rates in excess of 140 beats/minute. All modalities of Doppler including color, pulse, high pulse repetition frequency, and continuous wave should be available. Tissue Doppler has been used in the assessment of fetal arrhythmias.

There are certain essential components of fetal echocardiogram:

Anatomic review	• Fetal number and position • Stomach position • Cardiac position
Biometric examination	• Cardiothoracic ratio • Biparietal diameter • Femur length
Cardiac imaging	• Four chamber • Five chamber view • Long axis view (left ventricular outflow) • Long axis view (right ventricular • outflow) • Caval long axis view • Ductal arch view • Aortic arch view
Doppler veins	• IVC, SVC, pulmonary veins, hepatic veins, umbilical artery, umbilical vein
Examination of rhythm and rate	• M-mode and Doppler examination

The process of fetal echocardiography involves, anatomic imaging shown in Figure 11.1 and the different views captured in imaging shown in Figure 11.2.

Step by Step Pediatric Echocardiography

ANATOMIC IMAGING

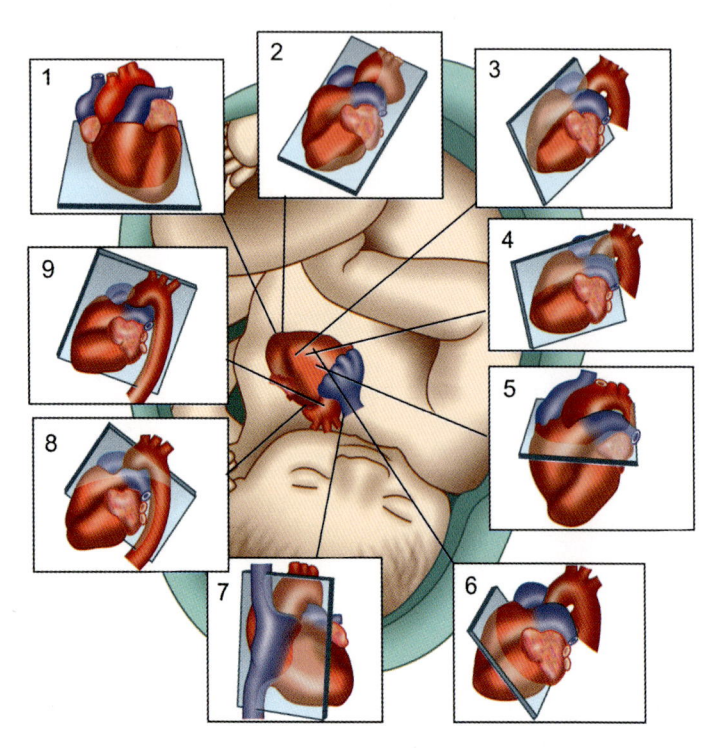

Fig. 11.1: Anatomic imaging. 1. Apical (4 chamber) view. 2. Apical (5 chamber) view angled to the aorta. 3. Long axis view of the left ventricular outflow tract. 4. Long axis view of the right ventricular outflow tract. 5. Short axis view at the level of the great vessels. 6. Short axis view with caudal angling of the ventricles. 7. Caval long axis view. 8. Ductal arch view. 9. Aortic arch view[4]

Fetal Echocardiography 121

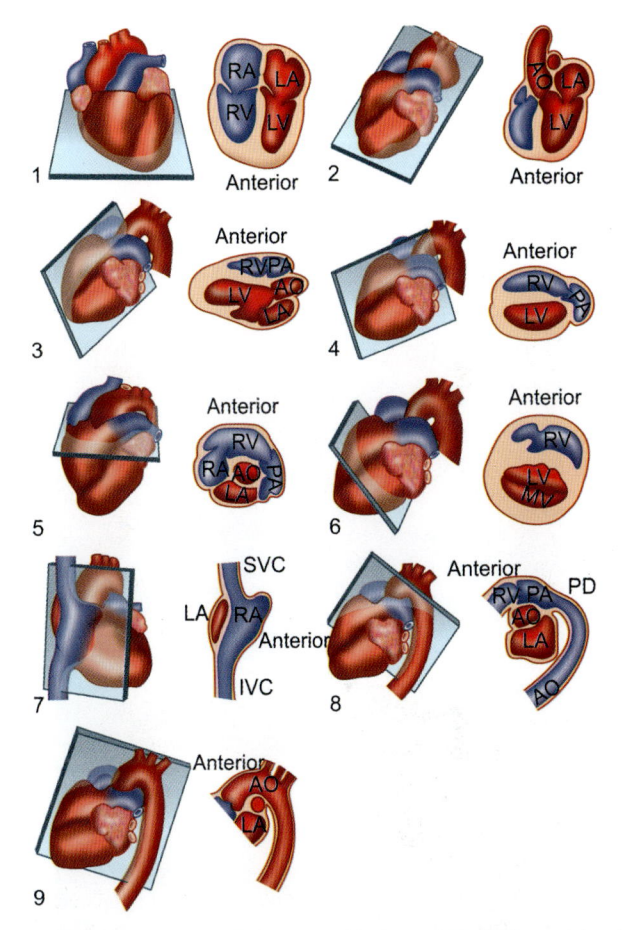

Fig. 11.2: Views and structures seen. Each numbered view relates to clockwise illustration of fetal heart AO: Aorta; IVC: Inferior vena cava. LA: Left atrium. LV: Left ventricle. MV: Mitral valve, PA: Pulmonary artery, PD: Patent ductus, RA: Right atrium, RV: Right ventricle, SVC: Superior vena cava[4]

Structures Viewed in Four and Five Chamber View (Figs 11.3A and B)

- Atrial and ventricular size
- Atrial and ventricular septae
- Atrioventricular size and function
- Coronary sinus

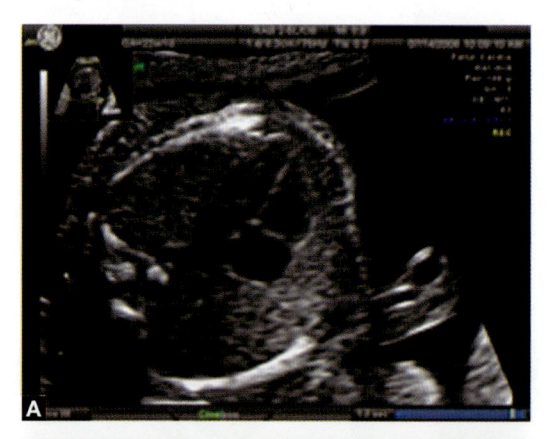

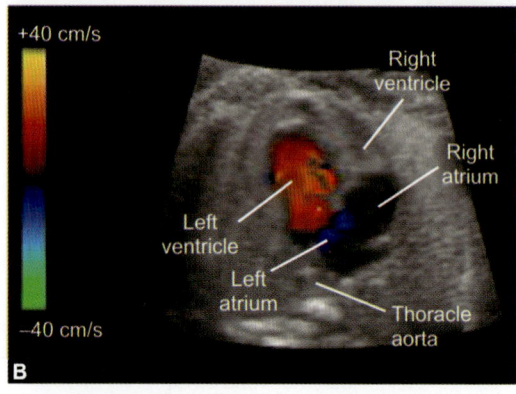

Figs 11.3A and B: Four-chamber view

Fetal Echocardiography

- Ventricular function in long axis
- Semilunar valve function
- Pulmonary viens.

Structures Viewed in the Ductal and Aortic Arch (Figs 11.4A and B)

- Main pulmonary artery.
- Branch pulmonary arteries.
- Persistent ductus arteriosus and direction of flow.
- Aortic arch dimension (ascending, transverse, isthmus and descending).
- Direction of flow in the aortic arch.

Heart Rate and Rhythm

- The rate and mechanism of rhythm is established by identifying mechanical events associated with atria

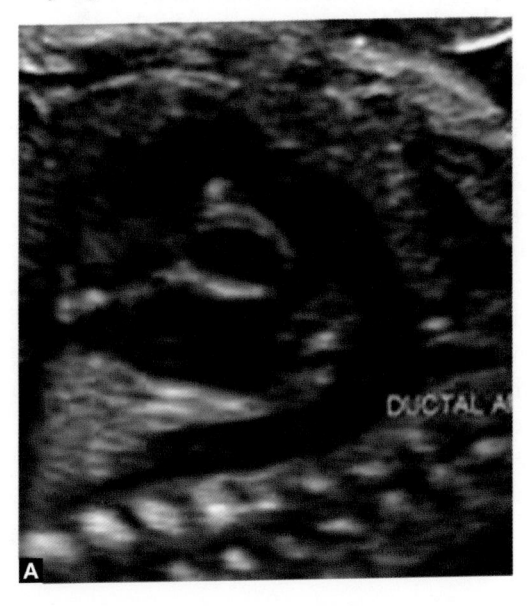

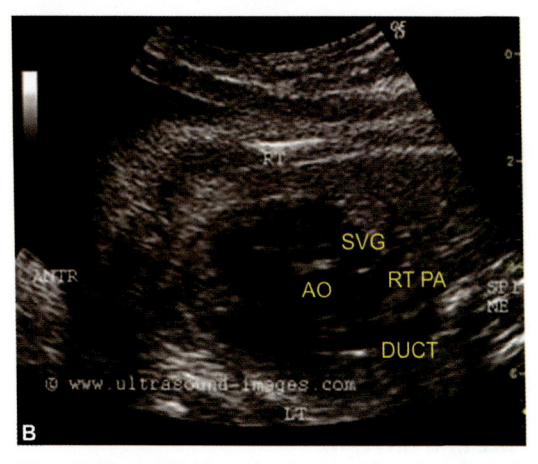

Figs 11.4A and B: View showing ductal and wortic arch

and ventricular systole. This is done by M-mode of the lateral wall of the atria and ventricles.[5]

Color Doppler Sonography (Required)

Color Doppler sonography should be used to evaluate the following structures for potential flow disturbances.
- Systemic veins (including superior and inferior vena cava and ductus venosus).
- Pulmonary veins.
- Foramen ovale.
- Atrioventricular valves.
- Atrial and ventricular septa.
- Semilunar valves.
- Ductal arch.
- Aortic arch.
- Umbilical vein and artery (optional).

In addition, pulsed Doppler sonography should be used as an adjunct to evaluate the following:

- Atrioventricular valves
- Semilunar valves
- Ductus venosus
- Umbilical vein and artery (optional)
- Cardiac rhythm disturbance
- Any structure in which an abnormality on color Doppler sonography is noted.

Cardiac Biometry (Optional but should be considered for suspected structural or functional anomalies)

Normal ranges for fetal cardiac measurements have been published as percentiles and scores that are based on gestational age or fetal biometry. Individual measurements can be determined from two-dimensional images or M-mode images in some situations and may include the following parameters:

- Aortic and pulmonary valve annulus in systole and tricuspid and mitral valve annulus in diastole (absolute size with comparison of left- to right-sided valves; left-sided valves measure equal or slightly smaller than right-sided valves).
- Right and left ventricular length (should measure equal).
- Aortic arch and isthmus diameter measurements.
- Main pulmonary artery and ductus arteriosus measurements.
- End-diastolic ventricular diameter just inferior to the atrioventricular valve leaflets.
- Thickness of the ventricular-free walls and interventricular septum just inferior to the atrioventricular valves.
- Cardiothoracic ratio.

Additional measurements if warranted, including:

- Systolic dimensions of the ventricles.
- Transverse dimensions of the atria.
- Diameters of branch pulmonary arteries.

Cardiac Function Assessment (Optional but should be considered for suspected structural or functional cardiac anomalies)

- Right and left heart function should be qualitatively assessed in all studies.
- Signs of cardiomegaly, atrioventricular valve regurgitation, and hydrops fetalis should be noted.
- If abnormal ventricular function is suspected, quantitative assessment of heart function should be considered and can include measures such as fractional shortening, ventricular strain, and the myocardial performance index.[6]

Complementary Imaging Strategies (Optional)

Other adjunctive imaging modalities, such as three-and four-dimensional sonography, have been used to evaluate anatomic defects and to quantify fetal hemodynamic parameters, such as cardiac output. Adjunctive Doppler modalities that have been used include tissue and continuous wave Doppler.

Ultrasound Safety During Pregnancy

The standard fetal echocardiographic examination utilizes all modalities of diagnostic ultrasound including two-dimensional (B-mode) imaging, Doppler and Doppler color flow mapping. Ultrasound energy expenditures increase with each modality used and are most intense when Doppler color flow mapping is applied to a small region of interest, as is commonly the case when examining the structures of the fetal heart.[7] Hence special consideration should be given to the ultrasound energy in the developing fetus.

As newer modalities such as Doppler applications assessing tissue motion and real time three-dimensional imaging continue to develop, bioeffects on the fetus will need to continue to develop, and monitored. As there are no strictly defined limits established, use of ultrasound energy in fetal echocardiography is best expressed as "ALARA" principle as low as reasonably achievable.[8]

The fetal echocardiogram is a unique ultrasound examination, which differs from the antenatal obstetrical ultrasound and from the conventional echocardiogram in the infant, child or adult. A unique high level set of skills and knowledge is required in order to perform this test.

REFERENCES

1. Hoffman JI, Kaplan S. The incidence of congenital heart disease.J Am Coll Cardiol 2002; 39:1890–900.
2. Carvalho JS, Mavrides E, Shinebourne EA, Campbell S, Thilagnathan B. Improving the effectiveness of routine prenatal screening for congenital heart defects. Heart 2002;88:387–91.
3. Stumpflen I, Stumpflen A, Wimmer M, Bernaschek G. Effect of detailed echocardiography as a part of routine prenatal ultrasonographic screening on detection of congenital heart disease. Lancet 1996; 348:854–7.
4. Journal of American College of Echocardiography. July 2004;17:806.
5. Kleinman C, Donnerstein R, Jaffe C, DeVore G, Weinstein EM, Lynch DC, et al. Fetal echocardiography. A tool for evaluation of in utero cardiac arrhythmias and monitoring of in utero therapy. Am J Cardiol 1983; 51:237–43.
6. AIUM practice guideline—Fetal Echocardiography, 2013.
7. Kurjak A. Are color and pulsed Doppler sonography safe in early pregnancy. J Perinat Med 1999;27:423–30.
8. International Society of Ultrasound in Obstetrics and Gynecology(ISUOG). Safety statement, 2000. Ultrasound Obstet Gynecol 2000;16:594–6.

chapter 12

Neonatal Echocardiography

Echocardiography on the neonatal unit has a high yield for the diagnosis of structural and functional cardiac abnormalities, often results in a change in clinical management, and can be a reliable tool in the hands of neonatologists. Utilizing the unique physical characteristics of the neonate and infant a simple reproducible technique has been developed which can be used in the nursery with a minimum of equipment. A minimum of five echograms are required for an "echocardiographic profile" of the heart and its great vessels. The profile consists of the quantitative parameters of the ventricle and atrial assesment, plus the assessment of the qualitative features of pulmonary artery-aorta, tricuspid valve-great vessel, and mitral valve-semilunar valve relationships as well as septal motion. The clinical application of this "echocardiographic profile" is very helpful in the differential diagnosis of newborns presenting in cardiorespiratory distress and/or cyanosis, rapidly separating those neonates with normal hearts from those with cardiac malformations. Its use in the abnormal hearts promises to make echocardiography a valuable tool for a fast and accurate clinical diagnosis of congenital heart disease.

Some commonly encountered problems like persistent pulmonary hypertension, ductal flow, atrial shunting, cardiac functions are discussed below.

PERSISTENT PULMONARY HYPERTENSION (PPHN) OF NEWBORN

It is most important to perform echocardiography to exclude cyanotic cardiac disease and to assess cardiac function. For this tricuspid regurgitation is important to assess. To do so pulmonary artery pressure (PAP) is to be determined. To determine this the jet of blood leaking through the tricuspid valve is interrogated with Doppler. The peak velocity of TR jet is a direct indicator of right ventricular pressure (and therefore PAP).

RV pressure = RA pressure + 4 × (TR jet velocity) 2.

It is important to determine the systemic BP to determine whether PAP is above the systemic BP.

DUCTAL FLOW

The direction and velocity of blood flow gives useful information of PAP.

Pure right to left flow indicates that PAP is higher than aortic pressure throughout the cardiac cycle.

Bidirectional flow occurs when the aortic and pulmonary pressures are equal. Flow is left to right during diastole and right to left during systole. (as the pulmonary arterial pressure reaches the duct before the aortic pressure waves).

Bidirectional flow is common in healthy babies in the first 12 hours but changes to pure left to right when aortic pressures become higher than pulmonary pressures.

ATRIAL SHUNTING

Some degree of right to left atrial shunting through patent foramen ovale is common. Pure shunts though this foramen, although rare, are diagnosed as Total Anomalous Pulmonary Venous Connection, until proven otherwise.

Bowing of the interatrial septum to the left is commonly seen.

Right to left atrial shunting reflects right atrial filling (diastolic) more than right ventricular systolic pressures.

CARDIAC FUNCTIONS AND OUTPUT

Elevated PAP is generally associated with decreased pulmonary blood flow and increased pulmonary vascular resistance.

Not uncommonly there is enlargement of the RV and RA, as well as main pulmonary artery.

There may be flattening or even bowing of the interventricular septum to the left if RV pressures exceed the LV pressures.

As cardiac output is dependent on the venous return to the RA and LA, cardiac output (both RVO and LVO) is frequently reduced with PPHN. Severe PPHN may be associated with LVO below 100 ml/kg/min (normal is 150–300 ml/kg/min).

Quantitative assessment of cardiac functions may assist with decisions and assessments of the roles of inotrope, inhaled nitric oxide, and other interventions affecting cardiac output.

If the LA and LV appear underfilled, it is critical to exclude TAPVD. TAPVD can be missed when assessing infants with presumed PPHN. Commonly in PPHN, RV is enlarged and LV is underfilled and squashed.

Demonstrating a left to right shunt at an atrial level essentially excludes TAPVD.

When the RA and RV are grossly dilated and the pulmonary venous chamber represents the confluence of the abnormal pulmonary veins draining in the systemic venous circulation which can be at the level of portal vein, coronary sinus, RA directly, or to an ascending vertical vein and then innominate vein.

FUNCTIONAL ECHOCARDIOGRAPHY

Targeted neonatal echocardiography (TNE) Point of care echocardiography (POC ECHO)

We should be able to perform and interpret TNE to rule out structural abnormality, also there is a need for direct measure of cardiovascular function, to see the effect of treatment whether medical or surgical and a need for serial assessments for various cardiac function and structural lesions like response of PDA to medical management. Last but not the least is the poor availability of cardiologists round the clock.

There is an increasing use of TNE in NICU since enough of theoretical informations is available and its utility is being established.

Indications

- Suspected patent ductus arteriosus (PDA).
- In a cyanosed newborn, suspected persistent pulmonary hypertension but necessary to exclude structural heart disease.
- The infant with heart failure, hypotension or shock.
- Newborn with heart murmur.
- Central line placement.
- Suspected effusion.
- Suspected thrombosis.

Components

Components of TNE are left ventricular function, right ventricular function, ductal shunting, atrial shunting, pulmonary artery pressure, measurement of blood flow and cardiac output, superior vena cava flow.

LV systolic function—Fractional shortening (FS). This is derived from an long axis or short axis, view M-Mode at the mitral leaflets tips with the beam perpendicular to septum is one of the most reproducible measurements.

Fractional shortening FS=[(LVEDD-LVESD)/LVEDD] × 100 LVEDD, i.e. left ventricular end diastolic diameter LVESD, i.e. left ventricular end systolic diameter. Normal values—Term babies 25–41%; Preterm 23–40%.

LV systolic function is also measured by mVCFs. mVCFs is mean velocity of circumferential fiber shortening mVCFs = mean [(LVEDD–LVESD)/LVEDD]× LVETLVET – left ventricular ejection time, from the closure to the opening of the mitral valve LVET. This is less sensitive to dimensional discrepancies.

Normal values—1.5 ± 0.04 circumferences.

LV systolic function is also the, ejection fraction (EF). This is the proportion of ventricular contents ejected during systole.

EF = [(LVEDD 3–LVESD 3)/LVEDD 3] × 100%. In this calculation any errors in measurements are cubed.

LV systolic function (SF)

Its quantitative assessment is an essential component of TNE. It requires the estimation of LV dimensions on the basis of M-mode or 2D measurements. LV end-diastolic dimension and septal and posterior wall thickness should be measured. On the basis of M-mode or 2D imaging, LV SF can be measured if there are no regional wall motion abnormalities and if septal motion is normal. In the case of wall motion abnormalities or abnormal septal motion, EF should be calculated using a biplane volumetric measurement.

Diastolic function

It is blood inflow causing ventricular filling velocities from four chamber view also the ratio of E:A wave E and A.

Diastolic function is blood inflow changes during the first week of life from dominance of filling during atrial contraction (A wave) to dominance of early contraction (E wave). Progressive increase of E wave and E/A ratio is more pronounced in preterm infants (developmental changes, diastolic dysfunction after birth?). Diastolic dysfunction, reduced both waves with dominant A wave. This is of no use in high heart rates with merge of waves. Normal values for term > 0.7:1 (E:A) preterm > 0.6:1.

Although the assessment of diastolic function and filling pressures should ideally be part of TNE, currently data are inadequate to permit any recommendation regarding the use of echocardiographic data in the fluid management of neonates and infants. Thus, this should be considered an optional component of standard TNE until further data sustain its use.

LV systolic/diastolic function is measured by MPI. MPI (= Tei index) myocardial performance index, is from adjusted four chamber view to get inflow and outflow. It combines the isovolemic relaxation and contraction times and corrected for the ejection time. LV systolic/diastolic function is MPI. It is less usable in high heart rates. It is influenced by preload and afterload. Normal values 0.25–0.38. Poor systolic and/or diastolic function > 0.38 ET.

The assessment of RV size and function should be part of TNE. Qualitative visual assessment remains the most commonly used technique in routine clinical practice. Two-dimensional measurements, including tricuspid annular plane systolic excursion and fractional area change, can be used for quantitative serial follow-up.

Atrial shunting is usually low velocity flow. In this color Doppler, pulsed wave is dominant shunting of left to right (up to 30% of right to left is normal). Pure right to left shunt is seen in congenital heart disease, pulmonary hypertension of the newborn (PPHN). Large atrial shunting increases right ventricular output, and decreases LA/AO ratio.

TNE should include evaluation for the presence, size, and direction of atrial-level shunting

Pulmonary artery pressure (PAP) is interpreted from ductal shunting and the ductal flow reflects relation of systemic and pulmonary BP. It is derived from color Doppler, pulsed/continuous Doppler. In suprasystemic pressure when right-to-left flow ≥ 30% of cardiac cycle, it is a R-L shunt. In bidirectional PDA flow is typical for first hours after birth, changes to L- R as PVR decrease.

TNE should determine the presence of a ductus arteriosus, the direction and characteristics of the shunt across the duct, and the pressure gradient between the aorta and the PA. The hemodynamic significance is further assessed by studying the degree of volume overload by measuring LV dimensions.

Pulmonary artery pressure (PAP) is interpreted from tricuspid regurgitation jet. Modified Bernoulli equation PAP = 4 × velocity 2 + 5 (atrial pressure). Most accurate of the indirect methods. 50% of a babies will not have tricuspidal regurgitation.

Estimation of RVSP and PA pressures is an essential component of TNE and is based on Doppler measurements of tricuspid and pulmonary regurgitant jets. The Doppler-derived pressure gradient across a PDA can also be used for assessment of PA pressures.

Left ventricular output (LVO)

Measuring of ascending aorta in diameter from long axis view, end-systolic internal (trailing edge to leading edge) diameter beyond the coronary sinus. Velocity is measured from apical or suprasternal view, average VTI from 5 cardiac cycles LVO = [p × (d2/4) × VTI × HR]/weight. LVO normal values—150–300 ml/kg/min.

Right ventricular output (RVO)

In preterm infants with PDA, RVO represent systemic blood flow more than LVO. Measuring in the main pulmonary artery diameter in low parasternal view, 2-D image at the insertion of pulmonary valve leaflets in end-systole. Velocity just beyond the valve leaflets RVO = [p × (d2/4) × VTI × HR] / weight. RVO Normal values 150–300 ml/kg/min.

Superior vena cava (SVC) flow

This represents blood from upper body. 70–80% is from brain. This is not confounded by shunts. Diameter is measured at parasternal view before entry to right atrium. Average value from maximal and minimal diameter. Velocity is measured at subcostal view. Average from 10 cycles SVC = [p × (d2/4) × VTI × HR] / weight. Normal values 40–120 ml/kg/min in VLBW.

TNE can include a measurement of cardiac index using the LV output method. In the presence of a PDA,

LV output measurement does not reflect systemic blood flow. The SVC method may be used to follow changes in cardiac output when a PDA is present, but caution is required when interpreting the findings.

Focused TNE can be used for identifying catheter tip position after line placement and potential complications such as line thrombosis or infection. Echocardiography to rule out vegetations should be performed or interpreted by a pediatric cardiologist.

Generally, a pericardial effusion is measured from the epicardial surface of the heart to its maximum dimension on 2-D imaging at end-diastole. Although there is no recognized standard for the measurement of effusions, measurement of the maximum dimension at end-diastole with identification of the location is recommended. For serial effusion assessment, consistent image projections should be used.

The ultrasound systems used for TNE should be optimized for imaging the neonatal heart. When imaging a potentially unstable neonate or VLBW infant, special attention is required for the prevention of infection, maintenance of body temperature, and monitoring of cardiorespiratory function.

Comprehensive echocardiography is indicated in neonates with perinatal asphyxia with clinical or biochemical signs of cardiovascular compromise. Standard TNE, including the assessment of LV function, pulmonary hypertension, and ductal shunting, can help in optimizing therapy.

TNE might provide useful additional information for defining the underlying causes and guiding medical management in the follow-up of hypotensive neonates in whom structural heart disease has been ruled out. Every child with a CHD should undergo a comprehensive echocardiographic study to rule out CHD and to assess the severity of PPHN. Standard TNE can be used to assess the effect of treatment on PA pressures, RV function, and shunt direction at the atrial and ductal levels. Focused TNE can be useful for line placement or in case of ECMO. NICU for this indication.

In every child with suspected pulmonary hypertension, comprehensive echocardiography should be performed to rule out structural heart disease. In neonates with PPHN, TNE allows assessment of the effect of treatment on PA pressures, RV function, and shunt direction at the atrial and ductal level.

BIBLIOGRAPHY

1. Journal of the American Society of Echocardiography. Volume 24, Issue 10, Pages 1057–1078, October 2011.
2. Skinner J, Alverson D, Hunter S(Eds). Echocardiography for the neonatologists. Churchill Livingstone 2000.

chapter 13
Echocardiography in Intensive Care Unit

WHY ECHO IN ICU?

1. Hemodynamic instability: It is the primary reason, when child is not responding to inotropes, despite adequate apparent inotropic support.
   a. Hypovolemia
   b. Pulmonary embolism
   c. Acute valvular dysfunction
   d. Cardiac tamponade
   e. Complications after cardiothoracic surgery.
2. Infective endocarditis or myocarditis
3. Aortic dissection and rupture as in Marfan's syndrome
4. Unexplained hypoxemia as PAH, CCHD with or without increased PBF.

PRELOAD ASSESSMENT: PREDICTION OF VOLUME RESPONSIVENESS

In a patient with shock, a complex interplay between preload, myocardial contractility and afterload.

A common problem we face everyday in management of pediatric patients who present with shock, is when to give another bolus in the presence of clinical signs of worsening shock, considering the complex heart. In this context, assessment of fluid responsiveness remains difficult, specially in hemodynamically unstable patients, whether it is cardiogenic shock or not, whether this extra bolus, will cause an increase in liver size or respiratory distress and tip the patient over the edge.

Mechanical ventilation causes changes in intrathoracic pressures, leading to variations in preload of the right and left ventricles, thereby affecting stroke volume and manifesting as changes in arterial pressure. Exaggerated ventilation-induced changes in the arterial pressure tracing are clinically related to the presence of hypovolemia, both in patients with preserved and in those with decreased left ventricular function. In septic shock patients, analysis of stroke volume and pulse pressure variation has been shown to indicate most accurately the presence of fluid responsiveness.[1,2]

Broadly the echocardiographic parameters in assessment can be categorized on the basis of echo measurements, with fluid bolus (either given extrinsically or generated within the body by means of passive leg raising).

Static Parameters

A static parameter is measured under a static ventricular preload status and is presumed to reliably estimate the preload of that ventricle. These include (left ventricular end diastolic area, Doppler mitral flow E/A ratio, pulmonary venous flow, tissue Doppler (E/Ea ratio), or color-coded Doppler (E/Vp ratio) static parameters appear to be poor predictors of volume responsiveness except in patients with relatively obvious hypovolemia.[2] Theoretically, they are supposed to be useful markers of volume responsiveness but few recent studies have shown, them to be poor predictors of volume responsiveness, except in patients with obvious hypovolemia. This led to evolution of more reliably dynamic parameters.

Dynamic Parameters

They essentially are for timed assessment of variation in cardiac function, in response to fluid shifts as during respiration or as an external source, as a fluid bolus, or by means of a passive leg raising test. It can determine, which part of Frank starling curve it is located on, ascending part, where more fluid resuscitation, can be of significant benefit, or in the plateau portion, whereby excessive fluid will not benefit markedly, and a support by means of inotropes may be considered. These include, bedside maneuvers such as passive leg raising (PLR) result in alterations of RV and LV preload can be utilized to establish similar correlations.

IVC and superior vena cava (SVC) diameter changes during mechanical ventilation, including distensibility indices, can be used to predict fluid responsiveness.[2, 3]

Transmitral parameters that have been studied include the ratio of early to late transmitral diastolic filling (E/A ratio), isovolumetric relaxation time, and the rate of deceleration of early diastolic inflow (deceleration time). A decrease in preload causes a significant reduction in the E-wave (early filling flow wave) velocity at the mitral level in conjunction with a decrease of the S-wave (systolic flow wave) in the pulmonary vein. In our daily practice in ICU, the E/A ratio is easy to assess. In conjunction with normal contractility of the LV, a low E/A ratio is usually a characteristic sign of inadequate preload. Pulmonary venous flow can also be used to assess LA pressure. A normal pulmonary venous flow pattern, demonstrating a predominance of flow during systole (S phase) compared to early diastole (D phase), will usually indicate a LA pressure < 8 mmHg, whereas the opposite predominance of flow will usually indicate an elevation in LA pressure (in the absence of significant regurgitant lesions [MR]).[4–6]

Septic shock has undergone a conceptual revolution. Earlier it was attributed to be a hypodynamic, low output state in association with myocardial hypoperfusion, now it is considered as a hyperdynamic, high-output condition driven by a complex interaction of circulating pro-inflammatory and anti-inflammatory cytokines, and cardiovascular adaptation to stress.

Some features are peculiar to cardiac function in septic shock, these include:

1. In early septic shock, systolic function is often impaired, with cardiac output being normal, myocardial depression may only become apparent when afterload is restored with norepinephrine.[7, 8] Impaired systolic function has been found in patients with low, normal, and even increased cardiac output.[7]
2. Approximately 20% of patients with septic shock have isolated diastolic dysfunction. Cardiac filling and relaxation are abnormal, whereas systolic function is preserved.[7, 8]
3. Septic myocardial dysfunction may reflect impaired adrenergic responsiveness, rather than deranged myocyte contractile function. Ejection fraction should not be used or considered interchangeably with contractility, because EF is influenced by preload. In contrast, most patients exhibited impaired adrenergic responsiveness, defined as a dose dependent increase in cardiac output with escalating doses of dobutamine.

PRACTICAL EVALUATION OF LV SYSTOLIC FUNCTION

The most common and important technique for evaluation of systolic function for ICU echocardiography is by visual estimate. Global assessment of LV contractility includes the determination of ejection fraction (EF), circumferential myocardial fiber shortening, and cardiac output (CO). The simplest quantitative approach is to measure the LV end-diastolic dimension and LV end-systolic dimension for determination of the fractional shortening (FS) percentage. FS is related directly to EF, and a normal FS is 30–42%.[4] *Also, mentioned in previous chapter*.

It is important to note that in the setting of regional wall motion abnormalities, FS may underestimate or overestimate global ventricular function and must be interpreted in light of what is seen in all of the 2-D imaging planes of the ventricle. Global systolic ventricular function can also be quantitatively assessed by fractional area change (normal value is from 36–64%) and EF calculation (normal value is 55–75%).

Fractional area change (FAC)
$$= \frac{\text{end-diastolic area} - \text{end-systolic area}}{\text{end-diastolic area}}$$

TDI Doppler

Tissue Doppler imaging (TDI) works on cardiac Doppler principle, but measures low-frequency, high amplitude signals of myocardial tissue motion as against the high-frequency, low-amplitude signals from red blood cells, used in classic Doppler. The apex stays relatively stationary, while the base of the heart is moving downwards, making a global twist, ejecting blood from the heart. The result is longitudinal shortening, radial thickening and circumferential shortening of myocardial muscle. Myocardial velocity profiles can be obtained in two manners: Pulsed-wave (PW) TDI and color-coded TDI. PW TDI is an online, live measurement, while color-coded TDI requires postprocessing of data. Peak systolic mitral annular amplitude and total excursion—as measured with M-mode echocardiography—correlate well with LV stroke volume and have been used as an index of LV ejection fraction. TDI defines the mitral annular movement and provides quantitative, reproducible information. One technique to quantify global LV systolic function is to measure the myocardial peak systolic velocities of the mitral valve annulus at several locations and to derive an average. A simple tool for the noninvasive evaluation of LV filling pressures is the ratio of transmitral early peak flow velocity (E) over early diastolic mitral annulus velocity (E') or E/E'. E' can be conceptualized as the amount of blood entering the LV during early filling, whereas E represents the gradient necessary to make this blood enter the LV. Therefore, a high E/E' represents a high gradient for a low shift in volume. European Society of Cardiology Guidelines have recently included TDI-derived E/E' in the diagnostic workup for heart failure with normal left ventricular ejection fraction. An E/E' ratio, is considered diagnostic for diastolic dysfunction, whereas an E/E' ratio, excludes diastolic dysfunction. An E/E' ratio in between 8 and 15 is considered suggestive but nondiagnostic for diastolic LV dysfunction, and other noninvasive investigations are needed to reach a conclusion.[9]

Diastolic Function in Shock

Diastolic ventricular (LV) dysfunction is associated with slow LV relaxation and increased LV muscle stiffness and influences stroke volume. In the ICU, there are many scenarios where factors influencing LV relaxation, diastolic distensibility, and filling pressures coexist. These factors may be linked to underlying disorders (arrhythmia, valvular dysfunction, pericardial disease, sepsis, and hypoxia), to patients' history (age, hypertension, diabetes mellitus, and chronic renal failure), LV diastolic function is traditionally classified into four grades primarily using spectral Doppler of mitral inflow and tissue Doppler of the mitral annulus.

In normal diastolic physiology, blood flow into the left ventricle occurs primarily during the early phase of diastole, resulting in the peak mitral inflow velocity during early diastole (E) being greater than the peak mitral inflow velocity of the atrial phase (A). The waveform of grade I diastolic dysfunction demonstrates E velocity less than A velocity as a reflection of impaired LV relaxation. Grade II waveforms are pseudonormalized (E greater than A) due to the opposing effects of impaired tissue relaxation and elevated left atrial pressure. Grade III waveforms display an E velocity much greater than A because atrial contraction is insufficient, in the face of an elevated left atrial pressure/volume, to propel blood into the noncompliant left ventricle. Tissue Doppler of the mitral annulus is considered largely preload independent and is a surrogate for the left ventricular relaxation rate during diastole. As opposed to mitral

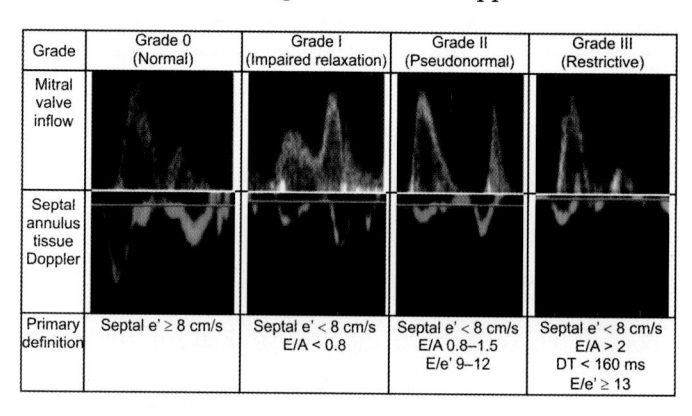

Grade	Grade 0 (Normal)	Grade I (Impaired relaxation)	Grade II (Pseudonormal)	Grade III (Restrictive)
Mitral valve inflow				
Septal annulus tissue Doppler				
Primary definition	Septal e' ≥ 8 cm/s	Septal e' < 8 cm/s E/A < 0.8	Septal e' < 8 cm/s E/A 0.8–1.5 E/e' 9–12	Septal e' < 8 cm/s E/A > 2 DT < 160 ms E/e' ≥ 13

inflow E velocity, the peak velocity of the mitral annulus during early diastole (e') demonstrates a monotonic response to worsening intrinsic diastolic function, with e' becoming slower with increasing severity of diastolic dysfunction. Moreover, the E/e' ratio has been shown to correlate with LV filling pressures in many patient populations, including those with septic shock.

Some reports suggest that the presence of LV diastolic dysfunction may be associated with poor outcome while others suggest no effect on outcomes.[10]

Right Ventricular Failure

RV function is influenced by conditions increasing RV afterload, that is predominantly lung-related factors, including high levels of positive end-expiratory pressure or increased pulmonary vascular resistance (from vascular, cardiac, metabolic, or pulmonary causes). Depressed RV systolic function is also associated with acute sickle-cell crisis, air or fat embolism, myocardial contusion, and sepsis. An assessment of the size and kinetics of the cavity and septum. The RV appears normally relatively flat. As it dilates, the apical region of the RV becomes more rounded. In the short axis, the RV (usually having a crescentic shape) becomes oval because of septal displacement and bulging of the RV-free wall. RV size and function are generally evaluated by visual comparison with the LV.

Measurement of Pulmonary Artery Pressure: The Dreaded PAH

A very commonly encountered situation is patient not saturating, with variation in SpO_2, with occasionally difference in upper and lower limb of SpO_2. Pulmonary hypertension, is one of the first things that strike our minds, it is quite common in the critically ill patient and is a manifestation of various pulmonary, cardiac, and systemic processes. It is characterized hemodynamically as a systolic pulmonary pressure > 35 mmHg, diastolic pressure > 15 mmHg, and mean pulmonary pressure > 25 mmHg (adult values. Systolic and diastolic PAPs are determined from TR and pulmonary regurgitation (PR) velocities, respectively (some degree of regurgitation is essential to be able to obtain a Doppler signal and subsequently determine PAP). TR is present in approximately 90% of critically ill patients. In the absence of pulmonic stenosis or RV outflow obstruction, peak RV systolic pressure is equal to systolic pulmonary arterial pressure.

Assessment for Intracardiac and Intrapulmonary Shunts

In critically ill pediatric patients, clinical suspicion for an intracardiac or intrapulmonary shunt is raised in refractory hypoxemia, when increased shunt fraction is suspected. In such cases, the presence of a right-to-left shunt needs to be excluded. Common origins of right-to-left shunt are atrial septal defect (ASD) or patent foramen ovale (PFO) at the cardiac level,[11] and arteriovenous fistula at the pulmonary level. A PFO is present in 25–30% of the normal population. Usually, a PFO only allows minimal and intermittent right-to-left shunting. When, RA pressure is raised and exceeds left atrial (LA) pressure, shunting across the PFO will worsen the hypoxemia.

In the critically ill patient, this increase in right-sided atrial pressure can occur from pulmonary hypertension such as seen with ARDS and pulmonary embolism, RV failure (from pulmonary hypertension), and from severe tricuspid regurgitation that is often seen in the ICU for a variety of reasons.

To be able to detect the presence of such a shunt at the bedside, a contrast study is often needed, as the shunt is usually not well-visualized with two-dimensional echocardiography alone. Color-flow imaging will somewhat increase the detection rate of intracardiac shunt, but usually only when the shunt is large. A contrast study should therefore always be performed when evaluating a patient with unexplained embolic stroke or refractory hypoxemia. Agitated saline solution is usually used for this purpose; it is a simple and easy to use contrast at the bedside. After injection, the contrast is seen in the vena cava, RA, RV, and the pulmonary artery. In the absence of a shunt, only a minimal amount of contrast should be expected to be seen in the left-sided cavities, as most of the microbubbles from the agitated saline solution are not able to pass through the pulmonary capillaries. If an intracardiac shunt is present, such as an ASD or PFO, left-sided contrast will be observed immediately after right-sided pacification and the contrast will be seen going through the interatrial septum. Performance of a Valsalva maneuver by the patient during contrast injection will increase the sensitivity of the bubble study to detect right-to-left shunting. In a patient receiving mechanical ventilation, a maneuver equivalent to a Valsalva may be performed by inducing sudden release of a sustained airway pressure previously achieved by inflating the lungs manually as in inspiratory hold maneuver.

This maneuver will reverse the atrial transseptal gradient and may help uncover a PFO that would not have been seen otherwise.

The characteristic of the intrapulmonary vs. intracardiac shunt is that there is a longer delay (three to five cardiac cycles) between appearance of contrast from the right- to left-sided cavities in the presence of an intrapulmonary shunt.[11]

REFERENCES

1. Usefulness of left ventricular stroke volume v... [Crit Care Med. 2003; May;31(5):1399–404.]
2. Levitov A, Marik PE. Echocardiographic Assessment of Preload Responsiveness in Critically Ill Patients, Cardiology Research and Practice, vol. 2012, Article ID 819696, 7 pages, 2012. doi:10.1155/2012/819696.
3. Charron C, Caille V, Jardin F, and Vieillard-Baron A, Echocardiographic measurement of fluid responsiveness. Current Opinion in Critical Care. 2006; 12 (3): 249–54.
4. Liebson PR. Transesophageal echocardiography in critically ill patients: What is the intensivist's role? Crit Care Med 2002; 30:1165–6.
5. Bemis CE, Serur JR, Borkenhagen D, et al. Influence of right ventricular filling pressure on left ventricular pressure and dimension. Circ Res 1974; 34:498–504.
6. Nguyen TT, Dhond MR, Sabapathy R, et al. Contrast microbubbles improve diagnostic yield in ICU patients with poor echocardiographic windows. Chest 2001; 120:1287–92.
7. Bouhemad B, Nicolas-Robin A, Arbelot C, et al. Acute left ventricular dilatation and shock-induced myocardial dysfunction. Crit Care Med 2009;37:441–7.
8. Bouhemad B, Nicolas-Robin A, Arbelot C, et al. Isolated and reversible impairment of ventricular relaxation in patients with septic shock. Crit Care Med 2008;36:766–74.
9. Van de Veire NR, Sutter J De, Bax JJ, et al. Technological advances in tissue Doppler imaging echocardiography. Heart 2008; 94: 1065–74. Accessed from http://heart.bmj.com/content/94/8/1065.full.html
10. Bouhemad B, Nicolas-Robin A, Arbelot C, Arthaud M, Feger F, Rouby JJ. Isolated and reversible impairment of ventricular relaxation in patients with septic

shock. Crit Care Med 2008, 36(3):766–74. doi:10.1097/CCM.0B013E31816596BC00003246–200803000-00015[pii].

11. Oh JK, Seward JB, Tajik AJ. The echo manual. 2nd ed.Philadelphia, PA: Lippincott, Raven, 1999.

Index

Page number followed by *f* refer to figure

A

Aortic regurgitation 88
   clinical manifestations 89
   ECG 89
      echocardiography 90
      X-ray chest 89
   natural history 89
   pathology 88
Aortic stenosis
   echocardiography 63
   features 63
   natural history 64
   supravalvular aortic stenosis 63
Assessment for intracardiac and intrapulmonary shunts 146
Atrial septal defect 47, 51
   clinical manifestations 48
   ECG
      echocardiography 49
      X-ray chest 49
   natural history 49
   patent foramen ovale 49
   pathology 47
Atrial shunting 130

C

Cardiac functions and output 130
Cardiomyopathy 101
Chiari network 18
Common atrioventricular canal 56
   clinical manifestation 57
   ECG
      echocardiography 57
      X-ray chest 57
   natural history 58
   pathology 57
Congenital heart disease
   atrial situs 46
   cardiac situs 46
   great artery connections 47
   segmental approach 46

Congenital left ventricular
outflow obstruction
types
subvalvular 62
supravalvular 62
valvular 62
Contrast echocardiography 9

D

Diastolic function 133
in shock 143
Digital echocardiography 9
Doppler echocardiography
29
continuous wave Doppler
34
frequency 30
pulsed Doppler 33
Ductal flow 129

E

Echocardiogram report and
its pitfalls 113
common difficulties 114
significance of a lesion
114
valves and associated
anomaly 115
source of pitfalls 113
assessment of pulmo-
nary artery
hypertension
115
related to machine 113

Echocardiography in intensive care unit 138
dynamic parameters 140
static parameters 139

F

Fetal echocardiography 117
anatomic imaging 120
cardiac biometry 125
cardiac function assess-
ment 126
color Doppler sonography
124
complementary imaging
strategies 126
equipment 118
heart rate and rhythm
123
indications 118
structures viewed in four
and five chamber
view 122
structures viewed in the
ductal and aortic
arch 123
ultrasound safety during
pregnancy 126
Flail mitral valve 88
Functional echocardiography
131
components 132
indications 131

H

Hypertrophic cardiomyopa-
thy 101

clinical manifestations 103
ECG 103
echocardiography 104
natural history 103
pathology 101
X-ray studies 104

I

Idiopathic dilated cardiomyopathy 105
clinical picture 106
ECG
echocardiography 107
laboratory investigations 107
natural history 107
pathology 105
physical examination 106
Infective endocarditis 93
clinical manifestation 95
echocardiography 96
history 95
laboratory investigations 95
pathology 94
Infiltrative cardiomyopathy
infective agents 111
Interatrial septum 11

L

Left atrium 44
Left ventricle
common measurements 41
diastolic function 42
global systolic function 41
wall thickness 42
Left ventricular output (LVO) 135
L-TGA
clinical manifestation 68
ECG 68
echocardiography 69
X-ray chest 69
pathology 68
LV systolic function (SF) 132

M

Measurement of pulmonary artery pressure 145
Mitral regurgitation 83
clinical manifestations 84
ECG
echocardiography 84
X-ray chest 84
natural history 85
pathology 84
Mitral stenosis
clinical manifestations 81
diagnosis
ECG 82
echocardiography 82
X-ray studies 82
natural history 83
pathology 81
Mitral valve prolapse 85
clinical manifestations 86

ECG 86
    echocardiography 87
    X-ray studies 86
    etiology 85
    natural history 87
Mitral valve-tricuspid valve 27
M-mode
    features 24

N

Neonatal echocardiography 128

P

Patent ductus arteriosus 58
    clinical manifestations 59
    echocardiography 60
    natural history 60
    pathology 58
Pericardial disease 96
    clinical features 97
        cardiac tamponade 100
        constrictive pericardium 98
        echocardiography 97
        quantification of pericardial fluid 99
        small effusion 98
        thickened pericardium 98
        X-ray chest 97
Persistent pulmonary hypertension (PPHN) of newborn 129
Practical evaluation of LV systolic function 141
Pulmonary stenosis
    clinical manifestations 60
    echocardiography 61
    natural history 61
Pulse Doppler 5

R

Restrictive cardiomyopathy 108
    clinical manifestations 109
        chest X-ray 109
        ECG 109
        echocardiography 109
    pathology 108
Rheumatic heart disease 79
Right atrium 45
Right ventricle 42
Right ventricular failure 145
Right ventricular output (RVO) 135

S

Standardized orientation of 2-D images 18
Stress echocardiography 9
Subxiphoid short axis 21*f*
Superior vena cava (SVC) flow 135

T

TDI Doppler 142

Tetralogy of Fallot 69
   clinical manifestations 70
   ECG
      echocardiography 71
      X-ray chest 71
   natural history 71
   pathology 69
Total anomalous pulmonary venous return 74
   clinical manifestations 75
   diagnostic criteria 76
   ECG 75
      echocardiography 76
      X-ray studies 75
   pathology 74
Transducers 8
Transesophageal 8

Transposition of great arteries 66
   clinical manifestations 67
   ECG
      echocardiography 67
      X-ray chest 67
   natural history 68
   pathology 66
Trauma
   systemic illness 112
Tricuspid atresia 72
   clinical manifestations 73
   ECG
      echocardiography 73
   natural history 74
   pathology 72

DATE DUE